MINDFUL EATING WORKBOOK

How To Improve Our Relationship With Food And Hunger, Stop Overeating And Take Care Of Our Bodies

JOSEPH RUIZ

Table of Contents

INTRODUCTION

Mindfulness is a Buddhist concept of meditation that helps you to recognize and understand your emotions and physical sensations. It requires focusing on the present moment as you acknowledge your senses, feelings, and thoughts. Because it increases your awareness, mindfulness has many benefits that can improve your relationship to food, other people, and yourself.

Mindful eating is the process of using mindfulness to get into a state where you have the full attention of every activity that you're doing. It helps you pay attention when eating. Instead of rushing the meal, you become more aware of the sensations and taste.

Mindful eating can help you feel in control of your eating habits. If binge eating, stress eating, addiction to sugar, or weight loss are a concern for you, mindful eating can help. It is also used to support conditions like depression, anxiety, and eating disorders.

Unlike diets or "eating styles", mindful eating doesn't require that you only eat certain foods and avoid others. By paying attention to what you eat, you may (as a side effect) reduce the amount of foods that are less healthy for you. Being mindful includes noticing what you're eating, how it is prepared, and how you feel when you eat it. Adopting this principle will adjust how you approach meals and snacks.

In this book, you will learn how mindful eating will improve all areas of your life. By developing this skill, you will naturally begin to appreciate and care for your body, your relationships, and your belongings. You do not need to diet. You will learn how you can embrace the practice of mindfulness and integrate it into your normal life until it becomes a core part of you.

How to Use this Book?

When dealing with any life challenge, it can help to reframe how you think. If you have a poor relationship with food, think of it as an opportunity for improvement, rather than a personal failing on your part. This opportunity can help you transform. By examining your biggest obstacle, you can gain insight and find the root cause of your challenge. You can become aware of your motivations and identify the various aspects of your life that can be barriers to making healthy choices. If you feel out of control around some or all foods, it is important to understand why you eat what you eat every day. It is also important to explore your relationship with movement and to learn what thought patterns, bad memories, and accessibility challenges there might be that keep you from nourishing your body with exercise. These insights will make you better equipped to break the patterns you have now and move toward living a healthy and active lifestyle. You will be empowered to make changes step by step and establish healthier habits.

Mindfulness can become a part of you. It will feel natural to fully enjoy every little activity you do in the present moment. You have a choice to live your life however you want. Seize this moment and begin anew. Mindfulness can be the catalyst for this process, as it reminds you to breathe deeply every day while eating breakfast, answering an email, or waiting in line. Mindfulness encourages you to take small steps and be persistent. With every passing day, you will feel more alive. You will find stillness in chaos. You will have a better understanding of yourself and your surroundings.

PART ONE

UNDERSTANDING MINDFUL EATING

CHAPTER ONE
WHAT IS MINDFUL EATING?

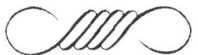

Being mindful is doing the same activities as before – walking, working, or eating – with careful attentiveness to what you are doing. Mindful eating is the practice of being mindful around food. All your senses are involved in choosing what you want to eat. You pay attention to your actions as you prepare your food, whether that is chopping vegetables or ordering pizza. You hear the sizzle of a hot pan and smell the fresh herbs. When you put food into your mouth, your mind is alert and present, rather than being distracted by the news, social media, or a conversation. You feel the texture of the food on your tongue and notice if it is too hot, or bland, or just right. After a few bites, you notice that the food doesn't taste quite as good as it did at first...or maybe it does! And when you start to feel full, you allow yourself to stop eating before you feel uncomfortable.

When work or an uncomfortable situation distracts you from your eating, you can reframe your thoughts to focus on your food. You might visualize the work that a multitude of farmers and laborers have done to get the food on your plate. Not only was your food planted, watered, and harvested but also had to be processed and prepared in a variety of ways to get to your plate. But even before that, the sun, wind, and rain had to cooperate to create the right environment for your food to grow. And before that, millions of microorganisms died to create a rich soil in which the seeds could grow. It is likely that, after considering all of these facts, you feel more grateful for your food and your present situation. You might let your mind get carried away with it, so just take a moment to acknowledge all of the energy, intention, and time that it takes to get your food on your plate. This is just one aspect of mindfulness, but it has strong implications that can help you reframe your view of how and why you eat.

A DIFFERENT PERSPECTIVE

Keep in mind that your body is not only yours. It comes from and belongs to your ancestors, grandparents, parents, and future generations. Even though you are your own unique person, you are also part of a grand story. Everyone has a part to play in this story. Having this mindset helps you to take care of your body because it can reframe your view of yourself. You might call yourself a caretaker rather than owner of both the earth and your body.

Eating Without Thinking

As you eat your favorite meal, what is always on your mind? When you eat while watching TV, thinking about a stressful situation like bills or a challenging relationship, or even reading a book, you are distracted from focusing on what you are eating. Food is most enjoyable when you practice *not* thinking too much as you eat. Instead, you can be mindful of what you eat.

Since your mind is not fully present in the situation, you may eat past fullness or eat something you don't really care for, just because you aren't paying attention. When indulging in a treat that you feel guilty about, you might dissociate in order to not feel as guilty. To be mentally present (and therefore mindful), you need to pay more attention to what is physically happening in your body.

MINDFUL EATING VERSUS BINGE EATING

Binge eating is defined by consuming a large amount of food in a short period of time, while feeling incapable of stopping when you're full. Binge eating can be triggered when you don't get enough to eat during the day, if you've had a traumatic experience, or if your brain chemistry is imbalanced due to an existing condition or medication side effect. Everyone binges occasionally, but if it happens frequently for an extended period of time, it is considered to be an eating disorder. Binge eating disorder's most visible side effect is weight gain. 70% of people who binge eat are considered overweight, and up to 30% of people who are trying to lose weight have a binge eating disorder. Mindful eating is the opposite of binge eating;it requires being fully present in the act of consuming food. In contrast, binging often involves a complete dissociation of the present moment while the body acquires as much food as possible. Practicing mindful eating has been shown to significantly reduce the severity and frequency of binge eating and can be a helpful component of treatment. It is always recommended to work with a qualified professional to support disordered eating.

MINDFUL EATING VERSUS EMOTIONAL EATING

Emotional eating is eating based on emotional triggers, such as a stressful conversation, work stress, death, or just feeling blue. Emotional eating is a normal experience that everyone has, but some people struggle with it daily.

If you feel "addicted" to food, you likely have a physical and emotional response to food that helps you self-medicate against another stressor. While emotional eating is okay to experience, mindful eating can help you identify when you are just eating emotionally as part of a routine, rather than coping with a specific situation. If you are eating mindlessly most days, then there is an unhealthy mindset regarding food that you can gradually shift with mindful eating. You can feel more in control of your responses instead of eating on a whim.

Characteristics of Mindful Eating

Mindful eating is easily understandable as a concept, but it can be challenging to actually do it. Here are the main characteristics:

1. You eat when you are a littlehungry, not waiting until you are ravenous.

2. You can determine if an emotional need is triggering your hunger.

3. You eat with as few distractions as possible, so that you can focus on all the sensory details present in the meal.

4. Your food is enjoyed at a slow but comfortable pace, so that you can identify when you are

satisfied.

5. You pay attention to what you are eating;where the food came from, where it has grown, whether it is organic or highly processed, and how your body will benefit from the food or be affected by it.

6. You can notice the effects food hason your feelings and your body as you taste, eat, and digest every meal during the day. You begin to replace automatic thoughts or reactions to food with more conscious, healthy responses.

CHAPTER TWO
UNDERSTANDING THE
IMPORTANCE OF MINDFUL
EATING

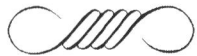

Who Can Benefit from Mindful Eating?

Mindfulness is a skill that anyone can benefit from. Just like meditation, mindful eating takes practice. It supports mental and physical health by bringing your attention to what you are doing in the moment, rather than allowing your mind to wander. The practice of mindful eating will guide you toward living a mindful life, and a mindful life is a peaceful one. Mindful eating reduces stress surrounding food choices, which can lower blood pressure and cortisol, improve digestion, and allow you to better enjoy and invest in relationships.

If you're concerned about your weight, you have probably tried dieting without ·lasting results. You may have gone from restricting calories, to cutting out carbs completely, to avoiding fat (or eating mostly fat). You may have tried juicing or other fad diets. And you probably lost some weight, only to gain it back within a few months. This is because any kind of strong, intentional caloric restriction causes your body to think it is starving. When you don't eat enough for an extended period of time, your body will rebound and send strong signals to eat so that you can stay alive. It is trying to protect you! The answer is not wholly on your plate. It starts inside your mind. Once you begin incorporating mindfulness, you will begin to understand that <u>food is not the problem</u>.

If you don't want to lose weight but still wish to feel in control around food, you can also benefit from mindful eating. You can learn to appreciate every momentinevery day that you live. You will appreciate food and how it nourishes your body. You can apply the principles of mindful eating to every aspect of your life when dealing withwork, sleep, and play. Doing this will support your health, peace, and happiness.

THE RELATIONSHIP BETWEEN MINDFUL EATING AND WEIGHT LOSS

If weight loss is your main goal, there is a larger mindset challenge that must be addressed. If you are someone who has wanted to lose weight for many years, you have likely tried many diets and/or exercise programs. They may work at first, but then your body attempts to protect you by slowing your metabolism in response. Weight loss slows or comes to a halt, and you become frustrated. You probably feel guilty and blame yourself for not getting it right. Every day is a struggle, and you wish there was a permanent solution to this problem. You are not alone!

There are many people looking for a magical weight loss solution. In magazines, televisions, or on social media, doctors, nutritionists, and influencers attempt to take advantage of you by marketing appetite suppressants, metabolism boosters, body shaping clothing, and gimmicky exercise machines. Countless diets emerge every single day with minimal alteration from the previous diets offering miracle weight loss. New research is published that contradicts health information that you thought was well-established.

All the while, you might be eating more energy than you need due to stress, mindless eating, or to cope with emotions. Over time, the extra calories build up and you might put on a lot of weight. Eating when you're not hungry day after day causes your body to store extra fat. Additionally, the current conveniences in more affluent areas means that a sedentary lifestyle is the norm.

Modern society has drastically reduced energy expenditure through daily body movement and opted for a desk job and dinner in front of the TV.

For those who are less fortunate, working 2 or 3 jobs may be required to pay the bills, and the stress of managing bills and schedules can cause mindless eating to be even more easy to fall into. Additionally, fresh produce is not always attainable in rural and some urban areas, leading to more reliance on fast food and convenience store food. This means there are plenty of chances to indulge in high sugar, fat, and salty foods.

The massive advertising in the food industry only fuels the fire. You may be more aware of the various flavors of soda and corn chips available than you are of how to create a veggie-rich stir fry from scratch. You may have adopted a habit of constantly eating and drinking, because that is what advertisers want you to do. Eating at your desk, in traffic, at restaurants, and while watching movies or TV are commonly accepted. However, it often leads to eating more volume than your body needs to sustain itself. And if your eating is emotionally led, you may not be getting the micronutrients you need for your organ systems to function, even though you have more than enough macronutrients and are gaining weight.

According to researchers, food that is high in sugar, fat, and salt can alter the chemistry of the brain and stimulate dopamine, which is a feel-good hormone. When enough dopamine is sent throughout your body, you feel relaxed and happy. Your brain needs dopamine to function normally. So, if your stress is high or you are going through an emotional situation, you may crave certain foods because they give a sense of satisfaction.

You may be wondering, what can be done? Is it possible to lose weight for good in spite of all these challenges? How can you be successful when there are so many ways you can fail?

Unfortunately, there is no magic solution. Most intentional weight loss programs are not sustainable. About 85% of people with obesity who lose weight tend to return to their previous weight, or a higher one, within five years. Intentional food restriction can cause emotional eating and binge eating, leading to weight gain even after successful weight loss. For this reason, many people who are sick of dieting have turned to mindful or intuitive eating for help.

However, it is incorrect to assume that mindful eating will result in weight loss. Mindful eating will help repair your relationship with food, which may or may not cause a change in your weight. Food restriction and/or binging will gradually recede as your mind comes to peace with food. If your body feels that its nutritional needs are being met and there is no threat of starvation, some gradual weight loss may occur. However, if your body naturally wants to be at a higher weight than it currently is, eating mindfully according to your hunger may result in weight gain. Trust the process and know that your body wants to protect you.

Your struggle will only get worse if you keep on doing the same thing over and over again. Changing self-harming thoughts and removing any association of food with negative emotions can help you improve your self-control and awareness.

Mindful eating can help you to live life fully and enjoy the present moment. Every second you spend worrying about the future and regretting the past is a moment you will never get back. It is a missed opportunity to engage in each part of your life and make positive steps towards achieving your goals. Live in the here and now and end your struggle with body awareness and confidence.

By being completely aware of what happensaround you from moment to moment, you can be more intentional about what and how you eat. You will learn how to stop your wandering mind so that you can concentrate on that present moment. This mindfulness allows you to experience peace and joy andexplore who you are. When you have practiced mindful eating many times, you will begin to see that your weight is much less important than who you are as a person.

The changes that mindfulness brings will require you to stop and reflect on the behavior that you engaged in that led to this moment. You will explore and come to understand why you're unhappy about your weight. When you look deeply into your situation, you will find a better way forward. Mindfulness is part of that path.

You will begin to recognize how mindless eating is a destructive habit and how to stop it. You can begin to accept where you are now and acknowledge how you got here. You can embrace the challenge and make a resolution to replace any behavior that does not serve you with behavior that serves your goals. You can be fully aware of everything that is happening to your everyday life, rather than ignoring issues that need to be dealt with. You can be in control and use whatever is within your power to begin to change. Only then will you begin to experience the change you want.

Mindful Eating Improves Food Satisfaction

Our society today has an abundance of food choices.

Eating is often mindless due to being rushed. Our fast-paced society makes us adapted to eating quickly. When you eat, it takes about 20 minutes for your brain to receive signals from your stomach that you are satisfied. These signals are activated when your stomach detects certain amounts of protein, fat, and fiber in the food that you ate. Eating too fast is problematic because the brain might not receive signals from your stomach until after you have eaten more than you need to be satisfied. If your meal had too little protein, fat, or fiber, your brain might never receive the fullness signals. This can lead you to feel hungry again in a couple of hours, or you might just keep eating until you're uncomfortable from the sheer volume of the food.

Rather than speed-eating, when you adopt the habit of being mindful, your attention is restored and you can slow down your eating. Therefore, eating becomes more intentional rather than automatic. It helps you know when you're full. Because of this, you become more in tune with your body's needs in general. You also can start to understand the triggers that would make you want to eat even when you're not hungry.

Once you can identify the triggers that make you crave more food, you can learn to respond appropriately to them. Eating mindfully means eating when you need to eat, not waiting until you are uncomfortably hungry.

Many people are so busy that they postpone eating until they absolutely must, and then feel ravenously hungry and overeat. If your schedule makes eating on a regular basis a challenge, being mindful will help you know when to start implementing strategic snacks or mini meals that can help you feel your best.

If you're on the opposite end of the spectrum, you might be afraid of hunger because it is uncomfortable, and you will eat to avoid experiencing it. This might be because you've experienced a time when food was not always available. Food scarcity is a major reason why some people overeat or eat frequently when not hungry. Another cause could be if your childhood involved poverty, physical abuse, or emotional neglect. The comfort of food might be one way that your brain is trying to stay balanced to deal with the aftereffects of that trauma. If you feel that one of these issues is a major cause of your poor relationship with food, you will likely experience better recovery when working with a mental health professional who specializes in the type of stress you've endured. Even if it seems like it is not a big deal, adverse childhood experiences have a significant impact on brain function and can make eating mindfully both especially important and especially difficult.

Mindful eating can improve food satisfaction by simply waking up your palate. If you've relied on junk food or monotonous meals in the past, paying attention to your response to food can help you identify your preferences, leading to the use of more spices, fresh herbs, and better-quality ingredients. If you were a picky eater as a child (or identify as one now), you might have limited your food exploration without intending to. Now is a good time to start trying new foods and foods you haven't tasted in ten or twenty years. You might be surprised in what you enjoy!

When mindful eating helps you increase the diversity of the foods you eat, it inherently improves your nutrition intake. This is because more variety of foods means that you are getting more diverse nutrients. All food sources have different vitamins, minerals, and phytonutrients that are needed by your body. If you've limited your intake to fast food, or only certain types of grains, or avoiding fruit, you've missed out on some important nutrients that food can offer. Not only will choosing better, nutritious foods help you feel more satisfied, but it can also help you reduce risk of many chronic illnesses.

Mindful eating can help you live a long, healthy life. It reduces the risk of diseases, such as hypertension, cancer, diabetes, and heart disease, all of which are associated with overeating. By learning to eat when you're hungry and stop when you're full, you will support normal metabolic processes that help your heart, liver, kidneys, and cells function better. By increasing the diversity of your nutrient intake, you will also be eating more nutrients that are needed to protect against these diseases.

Mindful Eating Reduces Stress Around Food

Eating mindfully can also improve your self-esteem. Overeating causes stress and discomfort and can infringe on your self-esteem if you have no control over your eating. Modern society, advertisements, and social media encourage internal pressure to have a thin, healthy body. If your body is considered overweight, you may experience bullying, social isolation, and self-harm as a result. You may turn down potential partners thinking you don't deserve them. Or your partner or friend may put pressure on you to change your body.

The pressure to change your body to fit someone else's standards can be especially overbearing when you feel like you have no control over your eating. When you eat mindfully, you're in charge. You are aware of exactly what your body needs, and you honor those needs. You can feel confident in eating because you know that you are not overeating or undereating. Your anxiety around eating begins to be reduced because you realize that the food was never the main problem.

You learn to enjoy the taste of nutritious food. You start to realize that some foods don't taste as good as they used to, or that some foods don't make you feel your best. You realize that stale, greasy, or heavy foods might not always be what will satisfy you. Or if you've been eating as healthfully as possible, you might realize that your body is asking for denser, hearty foods because you've been eating too many salads. As a result of the new awareness, your confidence in food choices will soar.

You will begin to sort out the emotional issues that you have around food. It may take longer than you expect, but you will gradually feel at peace with food. You will be able to eat socially without anxiety or mindless overeating, and you'll still be able to enjoy your food. You will learn how food affects your mood throughout the day. You will learn what foods fuel your energy and what foods slow you down. Then you can make more informed choices day by day. Eventually, you will be eating mindfully without having to focus on it so much.

Mindful eating is a skill that you have to develop over time with continuous practice. You need perseverance because there are times that you will forget to practice it. Don't give up! You will become experienced at it with time.

CHAPTER THREE
A GUIDE TO MINDFUL EATING

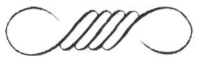

Choose Foods That Have the Nutrients You Need

Food provides the body with the right raw materials that it needs to run the metabolic processes required to keep the body alive. Most foods contain macronutrients; carbohydrates, proteins, and fats. Some contain all the macronutrients while others have one or two. The macronutrients have various functions in the body.

Carbohydrates' main role is to provide energy for the body. This form of energy is fast and usable by every cell in the body. Proteins provide the building blocks of tissues and organs like the muscles, liver, and heart. They also form enzymes that engage in cellular mechanisms like digestion. Fats form part of the cellular membranes of every cell and form hormones. They help the insulation of the body.

In food, we also get micronutrients, such as vitamins and minerals. These nutrients help to build tissues and catalyze chemical reactions in the body.

All these nutrients are essential to have a healthy life and prevent diseases. However, some nutrients in excess contribute to various diseases. For example, eating too many carbohydrates can cause metabolic inflexibility, which can result in chronic diseases like diabetes and hypertension. Therefore, knowing the right balance of nutrients to enjoy is very important.

The type of carbohydrate, fat, or protein you choose has an impact on your health. For instance, carbohydrates are available both in whole and processed foods, but not all carbs are equal. Whole food carbohydrates are available in unprocessed foods like whole grains, legumes, vegetables, and fruits. Processed carbohydrates are present in bread, pasta, sugary drinks, juice, and refined grain products like muffins and biscuits.

Unprocessed foods like whole fruits, grains, and vegetables are good sources of healthy carbs. They are also rich in fiber, vitamins, and minerals. Whole grains contain B vitamins and Vitamin E, magnesium, and selenium. Eating whole grain foods reduces your risk of diabetes, heart diseases, and cancer. The fiber present in these foods offers protection from high blood sugar. It slows down digestion after a meal and causes a gentle rise in blood sugar; therefore, it is good for controlling blood sugar levels. This is something you can notice when eating mindfully: if you are hungry within a couple hours of eating, you may not have had enough fiber or your processed carbohydrate intake may have been high enough to cause a high rise in blood sugar. When your body finishes processing the meal, your blood sugar may drop rapidly and you may feel hungry, fatigued, or mentally foggy a few hours later.

When choosing proteins, the type also matters. The most nutritious source of protein is in plant and some animal sources. Whole food plant protein sources include lentils, chickpeas, beans, nuts, and whole grains. They contain fiber, minerals, healthy fats, and vitamins. You may also enjoy vegan protein powder, tempeh or tofu, although these are moderately processed to increase the protein content. If you prefer plant sources of protein, variety matters because plant proteins are incomplete; they lack one or more essential amino acids. To benefit from a plant-based diet, ensure that you eat a variety of plant proteins to get all the essential amino acids required for body functions. This will also ensure that you are getting diverse micronutrients.

Animal protein sources are complete because they contain all the essential amino acids required forth body.

Some healthy animal sources include chicken, fish, lamb, grass-fed beef, eggs, and yogurt from grass-fed cows. Most red meat from beef or lamb contains saturated fatty acids that increase the risk of diseases like cancer and hypertension. When possible, choose animal proteins from a local source that moderates the food quality and processing of the animals. This is a good way to ensure that you are getting fresh, high quality animal protein. It also supports animal welfare by encouraging the responsible raising of animals for food. Additionally, cows and chickens that are raised locally tend to have higher amounts of omega 3s in their meat and eggs.

For fats, quality matters more than quantity. Some fats increase inflammatory signals in the body, while others activate beneficial hormone pathways. Healthy fats from plant-based foods include polyunsaturated fats and monounsaturated fats. They are liquid at room temperature unless they are processed to be more stable. They can be found in olive oil, avocado oil, nuts such as almonds, and seeds such as pumpkin seeds.

Omega 3 fat is a special kind of polyunsaturated fat that is found in high amounts in oily fish such as salmon. It is present in small amounts in grass-fed beef, eggs from chickens fed flax seeds, leafy greens, raspberries, chia seeds, flax seeds, hemp seeds, and algae. Omega 3 fats are especially important for your cells to function normally, especially in your brain and digestive system.

Saturated fats and trans fats are unhealthy fats that can cause illnesses, and they tend to be solid at room temperature. Animal-based foods like meat and dairy contain mostly saturated fats. However, the most health-damaging fats are trans fats, which are found in hydrogenated vegetable oils such as margarine and many convenience foods. These fats are chemically processed to make them solid and stable at room temperature, but they are incredibly difficult for your body to process and are often rancid, causing cellular dysfunction.

The type of fats you eat has major effects on your health. Eating monounsaturated and polyunsaturated fats can reduce harmful LDL cholesterol and raised beneficial HDL cholesterol. On the other hand, saturated fats have been linked to the rise of harmful LDL cholesterol and increased risk of heart disease. Trans fats also raise LDL and reduce HDL cholesterol, and cause damage to the cells in your arteries. They trigger inflammation, which increases the risk of heart diseases, stroke, and diabetes.

Saturated fats are difficult to avoid completely, since even healthy foods like nuts and olive oil contain some small amount of saturated fats. A good guideline to remember is to eat fats from whole food sources, avoiding saturated and trans fats when possible.

In addition to understanding how macronutrients fuel and affect you, it is important to know why fruits and vegetables are so beneficial. Eating more vegetables and whole fruits lowers your risk of high blood pressure, heart disease, diabetes, and increases your longevity. Fruits and vegetables are nutrient-dense, despite not being very calorie-dense. This means that they are a great way to get lots of nutrients without consuming more energy than you need.

Some of the nutrients in fruits and veggies are:

Vitamins - Vitamin E and Vitamin C boost immunity and prevent cellular damage caused by free radicals.

Minerals - Potassium lowers blood pressure and magnesium supports muscle function as well as control of blood glucose.

Fiber - These non-digestible carbohydrates fuel your gut microbiome, promoting nutrient absorption, fat metabolism, and disease prevention.

Phytochemicals - Non-vitamin antioxidants like lycopene in tomatoes and watermelons can protect against cancer, improve cellular function, and promote healthy metabolism.

Choose a variety of vegetables and fruits with

different colors each day to get these benefits. Include dark green vegetables like broccoli and kale, yellow-orange like sweet potato and carrots, and red like tomatoes and watermelon. Also add white veggies like garlic and cauliflower and purple-blue like beets and blueberries.

An easy goal is to consume at least five servings of vegetables every day. More is better! One serving is a half-cup of cooked or a whole cup of raw veggies. To get more, fill half of your plate with vegetables at lunch and dinner.

For fruits, ensure that you get whole fruits and not fruit juice. Fruit juice is high in sugar and lacks the fiber that is contained in the whole fruit. When possible, pick organic fruits and vegetables from the local farmer's market to get them at the peak of their freshness.

Hydrate to Satisfy Your Cells

Your body is comprised of about 70% water, primarily within and in between your cells. The more hydrated you are, the better your cells can function. This means better communication in your brain, better metabolic efficiency, and improved organ function. Water is the best thing you can drink, and it's necessary for good health. Most people start the day dehydrated from cellular detoxification during sleep, so it's a good idea to drink a large glass of water as soon as you rise. This can also help offset the dehydration effect of any caffeinated drinks you consume.

As you strive to increase your water intake, you can practice mindfulness by noticing how you feel before, during, and after drinking water. Part of mindfulness is knowing how what you take in will affect you. After you've established good hydration habits, a good mindfulness check up is to write down how much water you drink in a span of three days and observe how you feel in relation to your water intake.

While other types of drinks are perfectly fine to have occasionally, remember that what you drink the most frequently will have the biggest effect on your health. Fruit juices, energy drinks, coffee, tea, and other beverages offer enjoyment, and they can also result in a reduction of water intake just because you don't feel thirsty. Keep in mind that juices and many other store-bought beverages have different types of added ingredients like artificial flavors, sugar syrup, or artificial sweeteners. Fruit juices, smoothies, and sports drinks are all high in sugar, and it is wise to be mindful of how much you ingest.

Eat the Amount of Food That Will Satisfy Your Body

It's a common misconception that eating less will increase your health. Many people assume that eating less is best, especially if weight or health are a concern. The truth is that food quality matters most. The concept of "portion control" is incomplete because it does not take into account the fact that your body's nutrient needs change daily. However, it is true that eating too much or too little will cause stress to your body. This is where you might opt to follow food rules, such as "stop eating after 8 pm" or "eat only 80 grams of carbs."

You might be afraid that, if left unchecked, your appetite might take control and cause you to never stop eating. The truth is, your body is designed to regulate your appetite without any conscious decision on your part. You may feel out of control if your food intake has been too low for too long and your body's inherent survival mechanisms kick in to save you, resulting in eating a large portion of food. You may also feel like you can't trust your appetite if you have any metabolic condition that alters your hunger hormones, making it difficult to know when you are truly hungry and when you are full. The more you trust your body's ability to self-regulate, the easier it will be to notice and prevent overeating.

The same is true for the opposite scenario. You may be so busy or stressed that your body's appetite hormones are dysregulated, causing you to unintentionally undereat. This can cause malnourishment and increased stress on your brain and metabolism. Using the techniques of mindful eating will help you identify when you might actually be hungry but are unable to feel it, so that you can begin to gradually increase your food intake to a healthy level.

Keep in mind that your energy requirements are different from anybody else and vary based on your muscle mass, overall weight, genetics, and level of activity. Therefore, there is no standard amount of calories that you should eat. Some people should have half as much food as others simply due to body size or energy output. If tracking your energy intake is important to you, consult a health professional to help you determine your calorie requirements. This is much better than using a generic app that does not take into account your unique physiology.

In order to be successful in implementing mindful eating, you will need to have a support system in place. An online community, your family, work colleagues, or a small circle of friends may be able to encourage you when you aren't feeling great about your food choices. Your support group can also help you ensure that your environment best reflects your goals, by surrounding you with wholesome food options and opportunities to take a break and have a mindful moment.

Be Aware of Foods That Are Potentially Harmful

While all foods are safe to eat, some foods can increase your potential for illness if eaten too frequently. When you are practicing mindful eating, you will come to realize which foods your body doesn't care for and which foods help you feel your best. The following paragraphs are meant to be informative, but not cause you to restrict in any way.

White bread, white rice, and white pasta have all undergone processing that removes the bran and germ. This process removes all the fiber and other beneficial vitamins and minerals. What remains is the starchy endoderm. Although many factories do fortification to restore the nutrients lost, not all the nutrients that were stripped away during processing are replaced.

Eating a large portion (the majority of your meal) of refined grains causes your blood sugar levels to spike due to the lack of fiber. Your body can quickly convert the starch in refined grains to glucose. The glucose is absorbed quickly, and your blood sugar levels rise. In response to this, your pancreas releases insulin, a hormone that helps your body store glucose and normalize your blood sugar levels. The pancreas can become overworked as it struggles to produce insulin to reduce these elevated blood sugar levels time after time. When blood sugar is quickly returned to normal by the influx of insulin, you may become hungry again quickly. Another common effect is for the blood sugar to become too low in response to the hard-working insulin, which can cause sleepiness in the afternoon or general fatigue after eating. Over time, the constant sugar spikes and crashes increase your risk of developing diabetes and metabolic syndrome.

One way to use mindfulness with food is to notice how your energy is after you eat. Check in with yourself 30 minutes after the meal and observe how high your energy is on a scale of 1 to 10. Then, check again about two hours after the meal. If your energy is high 30 minutes after the meal, but extremely low two hours later, it's likely that your blood sugar has dropped in response to too much refined food. There are other ways this effect can happen, but low blood sugar is the most common.

Another thing to consider when selecting foods is the sodium content. Although sodium is an important nutrient, you may consume more sodium than your body requires. If you eat out frequently, salt your food heavily, or consume lots of food from packages, it is likely that you are over consuming sodium. High sodium diets are related to high blood pressure, and excessive sodium can contribute to dehydration if the amount of water you consume is not balanced according to your sodium intake.

Lowering your sodium intake can reduce your blood pressure, reduce the risk of cardiovascular diseases, and improve your metabolic function. If you have no existing medical diagnoses, you can eat about 2,300mg per day, which equals to one teaspoon of salt. If you have high blood pressure or have a risk of high blood pressure, it is recommended to limit your salt intake to less than 1500mg per day. This can vary according to what types of food you eat, how much water you drink, your activity level, and your medication list. Work with a qualified nutritionist if this is a concern for you.

It is easy to reduce your intake of sodium if you reduce the amount of processed foods you eat. In addition to the refined grains mentioned above, foods that are ready to eat often contain lots of sodium. These include frozen meals, soups, fast food, restaurant food, and processed cheese, as these have added sodium to improve texture, extend shelf life, and prompt your taste buds to want more.

Another potentially harmful food is alcohol. Although moderate consumption (2-3 drinks a week) of alcohol can reduce the risk of heart disease and diabetes, don't let this be the reason you choose to indulge. The risk of alcohol consumption outweighs the benefits. Excessive alcohol consumption increases your risk of hypertension, breast and colon cancer, and cirrhosis of the liver.

Alcohol is addictive and can be a barrier to mindfulness if it is inhibiting your prefrontal cortex. Practice mindful consumption not just for the benefit of yourself but your family and the community around you. Remember that how you live your life can affect others and your future generations. It can create a strong negative social effect on your family and community when you depend on alcohol to numb negative emotions. It is best to be mindful when drinking around children, since they are heavily influenced by your behaviors. How you treat alcohol can have a big impact on their future relationship with it.

Mindfulness will help you think of how your actions affect others. If you want to drink, ask yourself what your reason is for drinking and what effect may occur to your family and community. If you don't currently drink alcohol, you can apply this concept to any food, beverage, or other activity that you use to relax or distress. If you do enjoy alcohol frequently, consider reducing your consumption by a third or more to improve your health and critical thinking skills.

CRAVINGS AND SELF-JUDGEMENT

Many people turn to mindful eating because they feel out of control around food. Even if your weight is considered to be "normal," you may have a problem relaxing around food due to fear that you will eat too much of the wrong thing. If you've done any restrictive dieting in the past, you may remember the point when you realized that continuing the diet was not worth the stress it was causing you, and that food pleasure seemed so much more enticing than sticking to your rigid plan.

If you've been a target of bullying, whether from your family, other children or adults, or from yourself, this process of embracing mindfulness might be especially challenging. This is because being mindful requires you to accept what currently is, and that may make you feel unsafe initially because your body isn't currently respected. Most people feel ashamed and have a fear of being ridiculed, but the truth is that those people who bother you are the ones in the wrong.

When you start to eat mindfully, you may notice many more bits of sensory information pop into your head than before. This is because you are becoming more attuned to your environment, more physically aware, and you are creating new neural pathways that allow your brain to sort out all of that information. At first, it will feel uncomfortable, annoying, or boring because you have to focus so much on it. In time, those neural pathways will become more ingrained and mindful eating will be a part your normal routine.

When this happens, you may begin to notice that your cravings for salty, sweet, crunchy, creamy, and other tastes and textures are related to your mood, stressful experiences, or health conditions. It is important to acknowledge this because many people feel that their cravings are out of their control (and therefore bad). Instead, you can begin to see cravings as information, data that tells you more about your current state of being.

Cravings can be caused by nutrient insufficiency, microbiome imbalance, and other physical issues. They are not strictly related to emotions. This means that you don't need to feel guilty when you honor a food craving! Your body may require something in the food that you are craving, or you may be using food to soothe because it is the most reliable option when you are stressed. This isn't a moral failing on your part, but instead information that can help you make your next decision.

The same thing applies if you are concerned about your weight. Many people blame laziness, apathy, or emotional eating for their weight gain. The truth is, there are many factors that can affect your current weight, including your genes, lifestyle choices, past stressors, and your current environment. It isn't something that you need to be blamed for, but instead an opportunity to reflect and understand yourself. Once you identify how your body came to be in its present state (weight, cravings, stress, etc.), you can begin to make changes if you desire to do so.

You should also keep in mind that your body will naturally find the weight at which it is comfortable when you are caring for it as best you can. Food, movement, relationships, mental health, and stress management all play a part in your optimal health, and your body may hold onto extra weight or refuse to gain needed weight if it thinks you are still unwell. Since you cannot force your body to gain or lose weight, you'll get further in your health journey if you focus on habits you can control that affect your health.

As you delve deeper into the root causes of your health, don't judge yourself harshly. Don't keep on rehashing the past, or let the past failures hold you back.

Instead, look back at what barriers you have faced before when you tried to live a healthy lifestyle. An unhealthy relationship, working more than you absolutely must, self-pity, or lack of preparation could have been the reason you were not able to continue caring for yourself in the past. When you know where you might have trouble this time, you can use that information to prevent the same situation from happening again.

Seize the moment and begin again. Embrace whatever obstacles you anticipate so that you can transform your life. Practice mindfulness so that you can become calm and analyze the situation without self-condemnation. Mindfulness will help you to focus on the solutions and not the problems. Once you look deeply into your barriers and recognize the underlying causes, you are already on the path of healing.

CHAPTER FOUR
LIFESTYLE FACTORS FOR
MINDFUL EATING

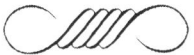

Mindful Movement

Do you exercise or move vigorously as part of your job? Government recommendations are to move vigorously for at least half an hour every day, or about 150 minutes per week. Having enough activity can help to prevent weight gain, but it is worth so much more than that. Movement activates hormone pathways that increase energy and vitality, reduce blood pressure, improve mood, and allow you to feel strong and confident. Even a small amount of stretching can give you some benefits.

Mindful movement is related to mindful eating, because movement helps you pay attention to what your body is telling you. Rather than retreat into your mind by playing video games or watching TV, movement requires you to engage in your body's sensations and appreciate the feedback it gives. This can improve your mindful eating practice because it increases your mind-body connection.

In general, the more active you are, the better your health. However, you may feel good doing just a moderate amount of activity, and that is perfectly fine. If you have a history of injury, chronic illness, or disordered eating, it is especially important to be mindful that your movement is appropriate to your body's needs. Work with a fitness professional or physical therapist to develop a movement program that best fits your needs.

Take a brisk walk five days a week, enjoy higher intensity body weight movements, or weight lift for 30 minutes each day. If you have been inactive for a long time, don't overthink it! Find some type of movement you enjoy and just get started.

When you sit down to watch TV, it replaces the time you would do physical activity. Watching TV may also encourage mindless eating, because it is easier to not pay attention to your fullness when you are entertained. Many people choose fast foods, sugary drinks, or energy-dense snacks when watching TV, which can throw off your sense of hunger and alter your metabolism. If watching TV is a frequent habit of yours, reflect on why you watch it. Is it because of boredom or stress? What can you do instead that can increase your emotional satisfaction and your level of activity?

Sleep Quality

Good sleep is a necessity. Every night, your brain gets to take a break from all the things it must regulate during the day and focus on healing and regeneration. People who consistently get less than 6 hours of sleep have a higher risk of many chronic illnesses than people who consistently get more than 7.5 hours of sleep. If you don't get enough sleep, you tend to be fatigued and it will decrease your energy. It also increases the hunger hormone, ghrelin, which can make it harder to choose foods that nourish you and may cause you to eat more food than you really need. When you stay up late, you may also tend to eat more than you would if you had gone to sleep a few hours after dinner.

Building a sleep routine and using good sleep hygiene can help you feel your best, but it also makes it much easier to eat mindfully. Mindful eating requires you to use your prefrontal cortex, the decision-making part of your brain. Until it is a habit, eating mindfully will take a lot of focus. When you are well-rested, your prefrontal cortex works much more easily. When you are sleep-deprived, it is difficult to do anything but the bare minimum and you tend to operate on autopilot. As part of your 4-week program, you will determine where your sleep hygiene can be improved.

DO YOU PRACTICE MINDLESS EATING?

High-speed living, coupled with the societal pressure and modern culture around food, can encourage eating on autopilot. You may not consider the portions you serve, how much food you eat, or even if you are hungry at all. Instead, most of your eating is likely controlled by external factors like the portion of the food at a restaurant, the plate size, or because you choose food based on your emotions. These are all aspects of mindless eating.

Mindless eating often leads to overeating, but it can also be used to describe not eating when you are upset, even if you are hungry or feel that it would be wise to eat. Eating a huge tub of popcorn as you watch a movie, having your plate filled for you at a holiday meal and being expected to eat it all, or sitting down for dinner after a long day and eating your food very quickly are all examples of mindless eating. When shopping at the grocery store, there is often a favorable placement of less nutritious foods that have a higher profit margin. And when you're at a restaurant, the perceived value of the plate is important, so portions are often oversized.

If you frequently eat in your car as you drive or at your desk as you finish that report, you are eating mindlessly. If you look down and wonder where the last bite of cake or steak or vegetables or candy went, then you are eating mindlessly. This is a completely normal part of the human experience, but it can also be harmful if it is how you eat most of the time. When you practice mindfulness, you can intentionally avoid some of these external factors that cause you to eat mindlessly.

YOUR WORK AND HOME ENVIRONMENT

Your workplace or neighborhood can influence your eating habits and lifestyle. If you have quick access to a grocery store, can find healthy convenience foods, and are able to cook most of your meals, then it is much easier for you to eat healthfully. However, if you live in a "food desert" (an area with no local grocery store), work more than one job in order to pay your bills, or have other responsibilities like children, pets, or an ill person living in your home, making time to eat well is much more difficult. If there are security issues where you live, and you can't run or jog in the morning, it may prevent you from being active. Think carefully about all the barriers to healthy and active living around your surroundings. Does your job prevent you from staying active daily? Do you get time for yourself and your family, or does your job keep you too busy? Once you identify these barriers, you can begin to work around them so that you make a healthier environment for yourself and everyone else.

FOOD AND LIFESTYLE PHILOSOPHY

Your attitudes and feelings can make you eat more and exercise less. If you impose certain concepts like, "I'm not an athlete," or "eating healthy food isn't in my budget right now," or "I'm just not into all that healthy stuff," you are probably limiting your potential for growth. Think carefully and be honest with yourself. Write all the negative feelings and attitudes that affect your lifestyle choices. Once you know them, you can work on them one at a time to break your mindless eating habits. Here are a few questions to get you started:

How do you feel about your body? If you could change one thing, what would it be?

What foods do you feel a strong connection to, whether positive or negative?

Who in your life has modeled healthy behaviors? What do you admire about them?

Is being a certain weight important to you? Why or why not?

Can you find time to work on your healthy behaviors? Or do you see no problem with your lifestyle?

What are some of the distractions that encourage you to live a sedentary lifestyle?

Do you feel that no matter what you do, your health remains constant? Have you now given up?

Is food what you use to fill the emotional void that you feel or to cope with loneliness? If not food, then what?

Where do you get health information that you trust? Is it from qualified healthcare professionals, social media influencers, or in magazines?

Do TV adverts influence you to grab a soda or fast foods?

Have you tried countless diets that promise to sort your problem out, but nothing happens, so you've lost hope that you will achieve your desired weight?

Do you have any preexisting medical condition that prevents you from exercising?

Reflect on these questions mindfully to understand what you can work on. The questions may be uncomfortable, but they will help you to know yourself better and help you to tackle the issues head-on. You will be able to focus on the barriers and motivations that drive you to practice mindless eating so that you can handle them once and for all.

IT IS POSSIBLE TO HAVE A HEALTHY RELATIONSHIP WITH FOOD

You have taken the bold step and analyzed the root cause of your difficulty with food. Because you no longer run away from it, you can direct your efforts to build a strong, healthy relationship with food that helps you feel amazing. Before you begin, it is important to assess your level of readiness. Ask yourself the following:

How would you feel if food never bothered you again?

How would you feel if your lifestyle was optimized to build your health?

What would it mean if you weighed more tomorrow?

What would it mean if you weighed less?

Are you ready to start today? If not, when?

You can be successful in implementing healthy habits, but you have to believe it. When you believe in yourself, you have the required faith to change bad habits and transform your life. What you believe, you can achieve.

Pledge to yourself that you will follow through with this personal journey to wellness. Create a mission statement which will remind you of your pledge. It might sound like: "I choose to take notice of every bite of food I eat, so that I can become more mindful and healthy," or "My relationship with food is important to me, so I am taking time to focus on it right now." Recite it wherever you can to give you fresh motivation and renew your zeal towards your goal.

When you begin your journey, it is very important to set goals that you can achieve. Whether it is to move mindfully every day, or to pay attention to what you're eating with each meal, realistic goals can help you actually achieve something and to know when it will happen. When you set these goals, focus on the present. Don't let previous failure and disappointments hold you back. Focusing on the present gives you the focus you need to change your habits.

Start with a broad objective, then refine it into specific, realistic, time-sensitive goals. The broad objective will remain constant for a while, but the specific goals may change over time as you improve and grow in mindfulness. Having big goals can overwhelm you, but if you use small individual steps, you will get moving toward the bigger goal. You will not get to your biggest goal right away; it will take some time and focus, consistency, and discipline. At first, it is difficult to change your routine. As you practice mindfulness consistently, you become more aware as you undertake your daily chores. Before you know it, it will become part of you.

You will become more joyful and at peace with your life. You will be in touch with all the beauty of life because mindfulness helps you adopt lifestyle choices that are good for you and the entire planet. Your health affects your immediate family and friends. It also affects future generations. You can contribute to the well-being of every person by being mindful about what you eat, not just for yourself, but for those who have not yet been born.

When you are feeling tired and less motivated, remember that you are the only one who is responsible for yourself. You can and must act for yourself if you want something different. Rather than blame others or shame yourself, choose to take this change seriously

Part of this journey is to accept your body and treat it with compassion. Rather than shaming yourself into change, use the uncomfortable feelings to prompt a close look at your lifestyle, and make changes that make sense. Don't be too hard on yourself. It is difficult to love yourself when you're just getting started, so begin with just accepting where you are now and be proud of choosing your next steps. It won't be easy, but a challenging journey that is worth taking.

While on this journey, give yourself attention, just as if you are taking care of a flower. If you stop watering the flowers or let them see too much sun, they will wither away and die prematurely. Likewise, give yourself the tender care and love that you need. You can use mindfulness to nurture yourself into the person that you want to be. It doesn't matter if you have had an unhealthy relationship with food for years, you can change it now. With mindfulness, you will learn to appreciate wellness and strive for it.

Take small leaps toward your goal. Don't set unrealistic goals that you won't achieve. It will make you feel like a failure. You don't need another experience of failure. Once you take little steps and succeed, you will taste the sweetness of success and it will push you toward more success. Even if you make just one change every week in the right direction, those are 52 habits you've let go the whole year.

THE DIFFERENCE BETWEEN MINDFUL EATING AND INTUITIVE EATING

You might have heard of intuitive eating, which sounds a lot like mindful eating. These two concepts share many of the same principles. However, they are slightly different. Mindful eating involves allowing yourself to be present when selecting food, using all your senses when eating food, acknowledging feelings about food without judgment, and being more aware of your hunger and fullness cues. It engages and uses the mind to concentrate on eating. You choose to eat in a calm and quiet environment by turning off the TV, so that you can engage the complete sensory experience of the food you are eating; the texture, smell, color, and how you feel after eating it.

Intuitive eating has many of the same practices but is more conceptual in nature. It involves listening to what your body is yearning for rather than what your mind thinks. It rejects the dieting mentality completely, as well as the concept that losing weight is beneficial. Instead, the focus is to make peace with all foods and to improve your ability to trust that your body knows what it wants. With intuitive eating, only a small amount of focus is actually on food. The rest of the time, you are deconstructing your internal stories about yourself and food, kicking out food rules, and rebuilding your identity surrounding food. It is inherently more political, as it addresses stigma surrounding socioeconomics, race, gender, and body size. It also encompasses things like self-care, movement, and activities that can give you pleasure and satisfaction that result in overall life enjoyment. Weight loss is not the goal. Intuitive eating gives you permission to eat what you want to eat and does not require you to be completely mindful as you eat. It acknowledges that mindless eating is sometimes part of an experience, and that experience can occur without guilt.

The similarity between mindful eating and intuitive eating is that they both don't seek to intentionally change the type of food or the amount that you eat, but they focus on how you engage with food, your body, and the eating experience. Both mindful and intuitive eating use a nonjudgmental approach to help observe and understand food choices. They help to reconnect you to your body so that you can pay attention to internal and external cues and provide a non-diet approach to heal your relationship with food.

Mindful eating helps you to get the awareness of how your food choices affect you and allow you to start noticing new things so that you pay attention. It makes you take time to enjoy the food experience and emphasizes attention to the body's cues of hunger and satiety. Mindful eating can be used as a technique to decrease how much you eat if that is what your body needs. However, you might find that you need to eat more if that is what your body needs.

CHAPTER FIVE
THE PRACTICE OF MINDFUL
EATING AND ITS BARRIERS

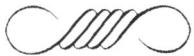

How to Practice Mindful Eating Every Day: The Step by Step Guide to Mindful Eating

We've already covered the basics of healthy eating. This next chapter will focus on how to eat mindfully. You will incorporate these actions into the 4-week program, but it is important to fully understand it first.

Mindful eating means that you eat with the awareness of every sip or bite when you are eating or drinking. You truly enjoy eating. You eat with compassion and understanding of the importance of the food before you. You can practice these steps with every meal or snack, whether you are eating alone at home or in a restaurant with other people. You can also practice mindfulness as you drink water on your desk.

Mindful eating helps you to appreciate the flavor and texture of food. It helps you to be conscious of the portion you're eating and the type of food you're eating. It creates a deep understanding of the relationship between the food we are eating and our health.

To practice mindful eating every day, it can be helpful to set a time for dinner and follow it like an appointment. Turn off the TV; put away the phone, magazines, or laptop. When you sit to eat, bring your mind and body there. Be fully present with the food ahead of you. Smile to yourself if you are alone and to others who are eating with you. Breathe deeply. Make a practice of pausing to breathe before you start eating. Breathe in and out a few times to be fully present as you eat. You need dedication as you practice mindful eating so that you can master it. Here are seven steps you can take to practice mindful eating

BARRIERS TO MINDFUL EATING AND HOW TO PREVENT THEM

Skipping Breakfast

The common fast-paced lifestyle makes it hard to find time for breakfast in the morning. You may have to rush to beat the traffic, get kids to school, or meet a deadline by 9 am, and choose to forgo taking the time to nourish yourself. Studies have shown that people who skip breakfast have a higher insulin response to food later in the day, which can promote reactive hypoglycemia, feeling sluggish after meals, metabolic syndrome, and diabetes. Breakfast is information: it kick-starts your metabolism after your body slowed it down during sleep. Eating breakfast supports normal metabolic function, gives you energy to power through your day, keeps you more satisfied with your meals, and helps you stay balanced with your eating. If you have been skipping breakfast or other meals so often that it has become a habit, you can consider these tips to help you change that.

First, prepare your breakfast and pack your lunch the night before if you won't have enough time to prepare it in the morning. You can pack dinner leftovers in your lunchbox and put them in the refrigerator so that you can grab it in the morning. Another option is to ask for help from another person living in your house. If breakfast would benefit both of you, make it a team effort!

Second, broaden the choices that you have for breakfast. You might be skipping breakfast because the traditional breakfast foods have become monotonous. Don't limit your choices. You can try different breakfast options like overnight oats, eggs and veggies scramble, yogurt parfait, hot porridge, or a flax seed muffin. To make it convenient and easy, prepare a batch to use for a few days. You can eat dinner's leftovers the next morning as breakfast if you prefer savory foods. You can also try breakfast ideas from different cultures: eat a burrito with beans, tortillas, or brown rice, tofu and vegetables, or miso soup.

Third, avoid overeating at night because it may reduce your appetite for breakfast the next morning. This is because your body may still be digesting, or because it needs about 12 hours to feel fully rested from digestion. Avoid snacking at bedtime so that you see if you will have a better appetite the next morning.

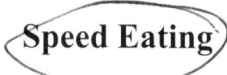 Speed Eating

Did you know that it takes twenty minutes for your brain to know that your stomach is full? And that's when everything is working properly! When you eat too quickly, it interferes with your body's ability to give you satisfaction signs so that you know it's time to stop eating. If you have a metabolic condition or have habitually overeaten for an extended period of time, your satisfaction signals may not be working properly. It will take longer for you to get the hang of mindful eating, but it is still beneficial and definitely worth it.

In order to help your brain, keep up with your

stomach. Eat slowly and make sure that you chew your food properly. Counting your bites when you first start eating is a great way to force yourself to pay attention and chew. When you eat slowly, you may eat less food and have greater satiety than when you eat quickly. Studies show that people who eat quickly typically weigh more and have higher risk metabolic issues than those who eat slowly.

To practice slow eating, chew one bite at a time and don't be ready with the next one on your utensil until you've swallowed the current bite. Think about every effort that has come together to bring the food before you. Notice the color and the smell of the food. Savor every bite until you finish the food. Take small bites and chew the food completely. A handy way to make this easier is to put the cutlery down in between each bite. You can also use small spoons to help yourself to take smaller bites.

Eating Large Portions

Most times, people overeat without being aware of what they are doing. You may eat too much because you eat out of super big packs or plates. You may overeat because you eat as you watch TV. You may also overeat because of other issues that don't have a relationship with physical hunger. Or, it could be because of the portion of food you are served in a restaurant or in someone else's house. However, the amount of food you put in your body is actually in your control. Your environment can make it much easier or much more difficult to eat mindfully.

To be aware of the portions that you're eating, use smaller plates, bowls, and spoons. This will help you eat a little less in your first serving. Wait a bit after you've finished the plate and decide if you are hungry or not for more food. Secondly, avoid distractions while you're eating: turn off the TV and put away your phone when you eat so that all your attention will be to your food. Take periodic breaths as you eat so that you can notice when your stomach is full. The breaths help you to relax so that you can fully digest your food.

Eating Too Much Food at Night

Most people who struggle with weight overeat at night. You make all the healthy choices with minimal portions during the day, but at night you can't stop eating. This is called night eating, where you eat large portions of food as you watch television or eat a large bowl of ice cream as a reward for a stressful day. Night eating could be as a result of waking up at night to eat or a serious disorder that interferes with your circadian rhythm, resulting in eating about 25% of daily energy intake after supper. This makes it difficult to be hungry for breakfast. If you suspect that this is an issue for you, it is recommended to work with a health professional.

You may also consider finding a hobby like knitting or reading to keep your hands busy so that you are less tempted to get food. You can also make it a rule to avoid eating as you watch television so that you are less likely to overeat unhealthy snacks. You will also likely see huge benefits from taking time to reduce your stress. Most night eaters have enormous amounts of internal or external stress. Listen to relaxing music or soak in the bathtub to unwind from a stressful day. Go to sleep early to avoid being awake too late. Getting enough sleep also helps to reduce abnormal hunger pangs the next day. It can also be helpful to choose fruits and vegetables to eat at night, because they are rich in fiber that will fill you up quickly. It is much harder to overeat these foods.

Eating Fast Foods or in Restaurants

Meals prepared away from home are often less healthy than home-cooked foods. Even the "healthy foods" served in restaurants aren't usually that healthy. The best option is a home-cooked meal. When you can't avoid eating out, consider these tips to maintain healthy choices.

First, before going out, <u>do your research</u>. Most restaurants have nutrition information on their online platforms. There could be menu options that have lower calories than the others, and this usually means there are more vegetables and protein present and less inflammatory oils. You can also just look for options that are high in veggies. Once the food is brought to the table, you will likely feel obliged to eat since you will pay for it. If the meal looks too large for your appetite, ask the waiter to pack some of it for you so that you don't overindulge. You can also order coffee or tea after your meal instead of choosing a dessert.

Convenient Foods

If you feel that you don't have enough time to cook at home and you prefer to buy takeaway meals, it's time to reevaluate your schedule. Your work and family commitments can make you feel that you don't have time to prepare food at home. But with careful planning, you can find time in places where you might be unintentionally wasting it. First, involve anyone in your household in meal preparation. Assign everyone a role, and in no time, you will have finished cooking. Or, if you live alone, pair up with your friends and assign each person to prepare one meal. Then, you can share them with each other and have some variety in your week.

Don't get into the trap of buying convenient foods to avoid making time for cooking. Convenient foods are often high in unhealthy fat, added sugar, and salt. Instead, make your food in large batches and divide it into small portions that you can grab for lunch or dinner. Prepare enough for the whole week and store some in the freezer for future weeks so that you have more variety.

Mindless Eating Trap Over the Weekend

Weekends are often the time where we get tempted and slip off our healthy eating plan. Taking time to relax and socialize may mean overeating for some of us. If you want to be more mindful, ensure that you eat the same on weekdays, weekends, holidays, and even when on vacation. You can enjoy whatever foods you like, as long as you are mindful of how they affect your body and take steps to choose foods that make you feel your best. It can be helpful to keep a food diary, whether for a day, a week, or a month, while you are starting this process. Keeping track of what you eat is a way to self-regulate and monitor your eating practices. Write down everything you eat, whether food or drink. You can use a notebook, phone, or online food log. You can even take a photo of every food that you eat. The more data you have, the more aware you will be of your food choices.

Another tip is to plan for your meals for the weekend

if you are up and about. Pack healthy snacks that you can eat on the go. If you will eat in the restaurant, check their menu online in advance and confirm the nutrition information so that you can pick the healthy choices. Another tip for staying track of your goal is to change how you do your social time. Instead of meeting for drinks or a meal, go for a brisk walk with your friend or go dancing.

EATING WHEN ANGRY, STRESSED, OR BORED

We have discussed comfort foods and the relationship between food and emotions. It may be easy to reach out for a candy bar after a stressful day. For other people, they struggle with eating disorders like bulimia or binge eating. Stress, anger, or boredom could push you to comfort foods. But you can change the patterns and stop emotional eating to stay on track.

First, practice mindfulness so that you can differentiate emotional hunger and physical hunger. Take deep and slow breaths before you reach out for food in your pantry, the refrigerator, or in the supermarket. Ask yourself if you're truly hungry or you want to use food to ease the stress that you're going through. Use a food diary to write down what you're feeling and the food that you eat when stressed so that you can identify the emotions that cause you to overeat. Keep tempting foods away from you at home or work so that you have nothing to reach out for. Replace the food with a book on your desk at work or keep a stress ball that you can squeeze when stressed at work.

Secondly, look for alternative ways to deal with your emotions other than food. Try going for a walk, doing yoga or meditation, or listen to relaxing music. You can try to talk to your friend or close family member about what you're going through. These food free alternative ways to cope with stress can be more sustainable than stress eating and will improve your health rather than degrade it. If you can't stop emotional eating, consult with a professional therapist who specializes in disordered eating.

PART TWO

THE ART OF MINDFUL EATING

CHAPTER SIX
UNDERSTANDING THE ART OF
MINDFUL EATING

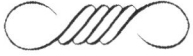

In the previous sections of this book, I have introduced you to mindful eating. You now have a glimpse of what it means to engage in mindful eating. However, there is more to understanding and identifying that mindful eating is beneficial. You need to understand that mindful eating is an art. As an art, it is learnable; for you to be adept at it and give your life a better meaning in relation to how you eat, you need to learn the art of mindful eating. In this part, I will take you through different methods and sections that will aid you to become a guru in the art of mindful eating. You do not want to live life without direction. I believe that the fact that you have reached this point in this book means you are ready for something great with yourself. It is a show of commitment, and in the subsequent sections, I will be taking you through how you can best commit yourself to become better at eating mindfully.

LEARNING THE BASICS OF MINDFUL EATING

One of the arts of mindful eating you need to learn and understand profoundly is the BASICS of mindful eating. The BASICS of mindful eating will help to bring to light the significant challenges you are likely to face with eating, and you will be informed on how best you can be transformed in your experience with food, which will also affect your body. Mindful eating does not possess any mystery whatsoever. It only has to do with you paying attention to the present and what is happening. When you fail to pay attention to what you do, you will look like you're on autopilot that only hovers around without specific directions. This will affect your understanding of the sensation of your hunger or satisfaction. You will end up unaware of what you eat, even to the point of not enjoying the meal. There is a war between you, your body and food, conditioned thoughts, and unconscious decisions. However, they are not the enemies. The best way to make novel choices that will honor your taste buds and health is to experience the present directly and recognize your thoughts and habits.

BASICS is an acronym used by Lynn Rossy, PhD in his book that provides the strategies for mindful eating.

With the knowledge you have about mindful eating, BASICS will be helpful for you to build yourself in the art of mindful eating. The acronym explains the best means you can take to be pleasant with food and your body, both at the point of eating or prior to eating. I do not want you to take these steps as rules; instead, they are guidelines to build a life filled with the practice of mindfulness at the table. When you give yourself to the directions of the guidelines, you will experience a significant change in your method of eating forever. The Acronym reveals the following meaning:

B – Breathe right and check your belly to know if you are hungry before you eat

A – Assess the food before you eat

S – Slow down the pace

I – Investigate your hunger as you eat

C – Chew the food thoroughly

S – Savor the food with knowledge

A. BREATHING RIGHTLY AND CHECKING YOUR BELLY FOR HUNGER BEFORE YOU EAT

Mindful eating requires you to give yourself to the

right breathing techniques and relaxation of your body. At first, take a deep breath and check your stomach. When you check your stomach, you are seeking:

1. if there is any sensation of hunger

2. the rate of your hunger

3. the specific thing you are hungry for

4. if there is any particular food you would love to eat

5. if you are thirsty

At times, a person can be hungry for other things which are not food, such as stretching, walking, relief from stress, and deep breaths. The general rule of mindful eating is that you should eat only when you are hungry. Most people breathe wrong and this holds some tension in the stomach. This is why it is so vital for you to check your breathing.

As you practice the right breathing technique, you need to place yourself in perfect relaxation. Relaxing in this sense requires you to take a few deep breaths, make your stomach soft, and permit the breath to be deep and full. You should pay attention to the differences in this form of breathing. Taking a few deep breaths daily will help you to deal with the habit of shallow breathing.

Breathing deeply is very essential to unlocking your body and improving your understanding, which will aid your recognition of hunger and satiety cues in the process of learning to eat mindfully. Breathing right is a good method for living a healthy life, and the most exciting thing about it is that it is free. You can always make use of it every time you so wish to do so.

AVOID SHALLOW BREATHING

You need to avoid shallow breathing as much as possible. To live healthily, it is crucial to avoid shallow breathing. There is a connection between stress and shallow breathing. The level of your shallow breathing will impact greatly on the level of your stress and anxiety. The symptoms of stress that a person is likely to have include muscle tension, rapid heartbeat, shakiness, clenched jaw, upset stomach, sweaty hands and feet, dry mouth, and having difficulty to swallow. When you experience these symptoms, it shows that you have been triggered with possibly the flight or fight response. There is a report that an average American is triggered with a short-term frame of stress response for an average of fifty times daily. This trigger starts immediately at dawn.

Stress makes use of the body's resources to avoid or prevent an imagined or physical threat. Whenever the trigger is activated, the response of flight or fight mechanisms can override your brain's ability to make appropriate decisions. The result of this is that you tend to be vulnerable to habitual behavior that includes you always reaching for food. The reason that food will become an option is that stress induces the secretion of glucocorticoids. Glucocorticoids increase a person's desire for food. Also, the insulin that aids in the intake of food is often induced by stress; hence, the propensity to seek out food increases. When you eat, you will reduce stress responses. However, it has reinforced your tendency to desire to eat. This explains the relationship that exists between stress and obesity.

The effect of shallow breathing does not just end there. The stress that it breeds in you further affects you. When you eat more as a result of stress, your body begins to store fat from the food. I believe you do not want to make your body a "fat bank". Well, it *would*-be useful if you have enemies you want to hide from. The fat stored in your body is converted to food when you need food later. It is a bodily method of creating a survival measure for you if you find yourself lost in the jungle and you need to hide from deadly animals. However, you are not a 5th-century hunter. Neither are you Columbus, who created interest in moving away from home. Storing fat will only sabotage the intention of practicing mindful eating. Have you ever experienced reaching out for food when you are angry, irritated, frustrated, afraid, or stressed? At that moment, the body is in need of relief from the tension that surrounds it. However, the food you seek in such situations can only provide a temporal solution. The unfortunate side of this is that when you go for food each time you are stressed, you will start subscribing to junk that you ought to stay away from while the problem that made you eat will still be present.

THE EFFECT OF DEEP BREATHING

However, life is so sweet and engaging. The interesting part of life lies in the fact that for every downside it portrays, there are always ways out of them. Deep breathing is what I call the situation that will take you out of the shackles of shallow breathing and give you sound health that will aid your mindful eating. Deep breathing helps to position you in a relaxed state void of stress, frustration, anxiety, fear, and any other unhealthy situations. You will be able to metabolize your food efficiently and still stay mindful. Deep breathing involves you breathing in more oxygen while you burn food properly. Each time you take a deep breath, the parasympathetic nervous system will kick in and reverse the symptoms of stress in your body. It will alleviate the desire for food. With deep breathing, you will realize the difference between the symptoms of stress and the symptoms of hunger.

CHECKING WITH YOUR BELLY

Checking with your belly helps you arrive at mindful eating. Each time you check with your belly, look deeply for symptoms, such as mild gurgling or grumbling in your stomach. These symptoms show biological hunger and your body's need for nutrients. Every time you ignore the sign of hunger, your body will keep speaking to you via other symptoms, including irritation, lightheadedness, stomach pain, headache, difficulty in concentrating, lack of energy, and faintness. From the symptoms mentioned above, stress and hunger seem to share the same symptoms. However, the source of their symptoms differs. The symptoms we get from stress are caused by feelings and thoughts, while the unavailability of food causes those of hunger in the belly. The ability to sense the difference between the two, however, is essential to practice the art of mindful eating. You should never equate every uncomfortable feeling in your stomach as hunger. Hence, it should not be fixed with food. Rather than looking for chips or chocolate, take a deep breath and look in to identify the message your body is passing across to you before you take a step.

I understand you may be shocked that you need to

check your belly before you eat since you are used to eating each time your stomach beckons you to. It is also possible that you are so out of touch with the symptoms of hunger that you have a problem understanding when you are hungry. At this point, it is expected of you to be skeptical about anything your stomach tells you. The untrustworthy feeling that you may have toward your stomach can be salvaged by mindfulness. Look into your stomach without being curiously judgmental and be kind. The care that you show is important as you improve your relationship with your body and as you engage in mindful eating. It often takes time, but your stomach will eventually become understandable to you. You only need to relax and start breathing deeply. Pay attention to the present sensation that you feel and ask yourself: "Am I hungry?"

HUNGER SCALE

There is a scale you can use to check how hungry you are. The scale shows your level of hunger and the level of your satisfaction. Using it regularly will teach you the language of hunger and, most importantly, aid you in the process of acquiring the art of mindful eating. The scale starts from the highest level of hunger to the highest level of satisfaction. Below is the scale:

Level I

Starvation

(You do not care about the quantity and quality of what you eat)

Level 2

Extreme hunger

(Lack of concentration, irritability, and other hunger symptoms)

Level 3

Hunger

(The feeling of the need to fill your stomach)

Level 4

Partial hunger

Level 5

Not hungry

(You are probably unsatisfied, and this is the least form of hunger)

Level 6

Satisfaction

(The meal seems to deal with your hunger; it is the least level of your satisfaction)

Level 7

Getting filled up with the meal

Level 8

Slightly filled up

(You become uncomfortable)

Level 9

Filled up

(You will be unable to eat anything, not even a bite)

Level 10

Stuffed

(The peak of your satisfaction; you are probably going to experience sickness)

HONOR YOUR HUNGER

It is a common attitude for most people. Many people are guilty of dishonoring hunger. Hunger is a legal experience. It is biological and, as such, should be tended to as you end whatever keeps you busy. Many people feel it is a distraction; hence, they are fond of denying themselves the need to fill their hunger. However, the first step you need to take to become adept at the art of mindful eating is to honor your hunger. Your body must have the sense that it will constantly have access to food. The result of dishonoring your hunger is "Starvation".

Moreover, hunger has a way of paying a person back for dishonoring it. When you starve yourself, you become like a wolf devouring whatever is presented before you without minding the type of food it is. The feeling you have when you starve is termed "Hangry" instead of "Hungry".

A person can dishonor hunger to an extreme level before it becomes starvation. At the Extreme Hunger level, you become unfocused, irritable, and start feeling some emotional disorders, which are indications that you have not had food for too long. This level is also not appropriate. Honor your hunger by eating at level three when hunger begins. At this stage, you may start having hunger pangs. It is the best time to sit and fill your stomach. If you give in to your hunger and start eating immediately, the pangs show there will still be the feeling of hunger at the start of your eating. That feeling signals that you reached level four. As you keep eating, the hunger will reduce while you won't feel satisfied, but not hungry either. This level is the least in the hunger levels. The next level you will reach is the level of satisfaction, which is where you need to stop eating. At this point, you have to give the best honor you can ever give to your hunger.

If you keep eating after reaching this level, you are already dishonoring your hunger again, and it will have an adverse effect on you. The next level will be eating too much, getting too filled up, and finally, stuffing up your stomach, which is providing more than is needed for your hunger. Each time you dishonor your hunger by eating when you are not hungry or eating much more when you are already satisfied are signs that you are practicing mindless eating. Such mindless eating is also considered engaging in unconscious eating or eating to satisfy your emotional needs. The hunger scale should help you regulate your attitude toward food.

IMPORTANCE OF CHECKING WITH YOUR BELLY

When you check with your belly, you access information on the status of your hunger and satisfaction. When you start checking with your belly, you will become more mindful of your eating. This will reveal to you that eating beyond your level of hunger need is not desirable and should not be adopted. Checking with your stomach will help you identify the discomfort you feel in your body when you reach the highest level of satisfaction before you stop eating. Identifying the discomfort should make you acknowledge it, and I want to be so sure you will not choose to keep experiencing such discomfort each time you eat.

Your body offers messages that demand to listen, understand, and honor your hunger and your satisfaction cues. It is possible for you to have little or no information on how you can eat mindfully by listening to your body, especially if you aren't used to paying attention to those messages before now. You will have challenges when first learning the art of mindful eating. It is possible that you will feel hungry most of the time, or you may never feel hungry. When you are faced with such feelings, what should you do? I will take you through the realities and the needed actions to take in such situations.

Reality One: One common occurrence is to have difficulty knowing whether you're hungry or not. There are many reasons for this. When you are unable to identify whether you are hungry or not, you may end up neglecting the other needs of your body, such as water, sleep, and movement. This feeling of hunger's death in you can be caused by the following:

- When you are used to drinking diet soda, coffee, and tea. All these can kill hunger. They are calorie-free beverages that give a temporal sense of satisfaction in the belly, and they knock off the hunger symptoms.

- Engaging in a diet for long periods of time. Most dieters who are fond of denying their hunger can eventually learn to tune out their symptoms of hunger until the pangs become difficult to recognize.

- If a person is used to eating according to the time. An example would be eating your breakfast at 7 00 a.m., your lunch at noon, and dinner at 7:00 p.m. After a while, this pattern of eating can increase a person's reliance on external factors, instead of internal signals to identify your hunger. Your ability to feel and hear your hunger's need will be dampened. If you plan to eat at a specific time, check your hunger and gauge the level. Mindfully eat the amount that will satisfy your hunger need.

- Living a busy life. This results in ignoring or suppressing your hunger to focus on other activities.

- Rumination. When you live more in your head than your body, the message of hunger can be shut off. Being lost in thought makes it difficult to practice mindful eating because you will not be aware of your hunger.

Reality Two*:* You may be feeling hungry from time to time. If you fall into this category, there are certain factors that you need to look out for. I have identified some of such factors. Look into them critically and identify the possible factor that may be contributing to your continuous search for food. They are:

1. When you eat food that does not possess the capacity to satisfy your hunger for long, you will end up needing food sooner than later. Most of the foods that fall into this category are carbohydrates, including pasta, sugary foods, and refined bread. These foods are easily absorbed into the blood; they help to increase blood sugar and insulin. Insulin prompts cells to absorb sugar

for energy or storage. The result is that the levels in the bloodstream begin to fall. Your body will start feeling the sensation of lack of fuel, which prompts hunger. Instead of reaching for nutrients, however, you will keep craving more carbohydrates.

2. Dehydration caused by not drinking enough water can expand your appetite for more food. Dehydration can mimic the symptoms of hunger. This is because the signals you have when you are hungry and thirsty are controlled in the same area of the brain. This makes it quite difficult in such a situation to be able to distinguish between the need for water or food. Make an effort to drink about sixty-four ounces of water daily so you can stay hydrated.

3. Your thoughts can be the reason behind your incessant want for food. When you think more about food, you will easily set off cravings. The thought will create a desire for food in you, which is not the same thing as hunger. You need to understand this early enough.

Nonetheless, some psychological, physiological, and environmental factors can make it demanding for you to check with your belly and evaluate your hunger needs.

You end up feeling more or less hungry. Just as I have mentioned earlier, stress, depression, and anxiety can make you feel hungrier. Also, medications can have an effect on your sense of hunger, either by reducing it or increasing it. Medications that lead to nausea, ADHD drugs, and certain diabetes' medicines can make you feel hungrier. You can be hungry after just smelling delicious food. The smell can get to a person's salivary glands and induce the urge to eat, even when a person is not hungry. The best method to utilize in learning the art of mindful eating is to eat when you are hungry and stay away from food once your hunger has been satisfied. However, there are specific situations when that may not work. This is the reason you need to become closer to your body and understand what it needs or requires. Your understanding of your body by being able to check in with your belly will help you identify when you need to eat. It will also help you know when you ought to stay away from food, even when you do not feel hungry. You should take a look at the following suggestions to understand your body better:

1. What You Eat Determines the Fuel of Your Energy

The foundation of your health is to eat what will fuel your body's energy. To keep your body actively working, you need to eat mindfully every four or five hours. At the start of listening to your body cues, this should be your guide. You don't need to eat a lot. Eating a little, such as a few nuts or a slice of cheese, might be all your body requires to stay fine until you have the next meal. You need to stay tuned to the symptoms of hunger consciously; you may not be able to recognize them at first and miss them.

2. Do Not Skip Breakfast

This is coming again. I have mentioned this earlier while I wrote about the factors that hinder mindful eating. According to research, it was reported that you need to eat more food in the morning, not less. You also need to prevent eating fatty foods and sugary snacks. Also, it has been discovered that when you eat breakfast mindfully, you will be able to concentrate more. Mindful eating experience increases alertness. Also, it reduces headaches and stomach aches. When you eat smaller food frequently and mindfully in the morning, it is equivalent to eating less over the course of the day and lowering your body index. When you skip your meals (especially breakfast), it will make weight control difficult.

Whether you are hungry or not, make sure you eat breakfast mindfully. That may be a piece of fruit, yogurt, oatmeal, or an energy bar. The most important meal of the day is breakfast. It is a good method of recalibrating one's body by jumpstarting the process of your metabolism, having not eaten for a period of time while you were asleep. It is most important that you eat something when you know you would not be able to eat for a long time. Make sure you do not starve yourself.

<u>Deep breathing and checking with your belly</u> are essential for you to learn the art of mindful eating. It will change how you eat and make you do it mindfully. It will also go further by affecting you personally and enhancing how you relate to yourself and your life. It also will help you discover hunger at every level, even when it is subtle. You only need to work with the practice. Patience is, however, the key in the process of learning to breathe deeply and checking in with yourself. Connect yourself to your body and listen to it through mindful eating. Having identified your hunger, seek what you are hungry for. You need to either investigate what your body wants deeper or have access to it at the surface level. To be able to do this, the next step you would take in BASIC will be helpful.

CHAPTER SEVEN
ASSESS THE FOOD BEFORE YOU EAT

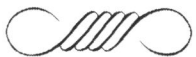

Mindful eating requires you to have the art of understanding the food you want to eat. Assessing the food involves you looking at its appearance, paying attention to the colors, and checking whether it is appealing to you or not. In the process of assessing, you need to activate your olfactory sense organ and identify the type of smell it gives. You could use Google Maps to identify where the food came from. You should be able to recognize the food; that is, is it processed or natural? Some food can be so processed that a person will lose track of what it is. Assessing the food should be with the mindset of checking if the food will serve what you want. Assessing food does not have to take a lot of time. A brief moment of assessment is enough to give you information. After the first assessment before eating, you need to reassess the food after some bites to ascertain whether your initial impression about the food was right or not. The decision then will show whether you need to keep eating the food or not.

ENGAGING IN FOOD ASSESSMENT

After having taken the deep practice breathing and checking with your belly, the assessment of your food is the next step. For many people to assess what they eat, they pick it up, throw it in their mouth, and swallow. It is a show of mindless eating for a person to eat without assessing the food. When you are engaged in mindless eating, you are only eating what you see because it is there. Before you eat anything, take a look at it twice, as if you are eating it for the first time. During your food assessment, you would have activated your sense of sight and smell to know about the food you plan to eat. Assessing your food does not necessarily involve your sense of taste. At times, before you start eating, you might feel your mouth beginning to water.

The purpose of assessing the food is to get a sense of how healthy it is by tuning mindfully into its look, smell, and how it feels in your hands. You should assess if your body would accept it or not. You may utilize visualization here by imagining it. You may think about this: what would it feel like for you to hold a cupcake?

What would it feel like for you to hold a bag of French fries? Identify the varying impressions that you get from different types of food. When you are able to do this, it will be easier for you to feel the texture, smell the odors, and sense the reactions in the body.

A HINDRANCE TO FOOD ASSESSMENT

Processed foods are a hindrance to assessing food. If you eat a lot of foods that are highly processed, it will be quite difficult for you to use your sense to assess food. The reason is that packaged foods are hard to smell, difficult to touch, and difficult to sense. Also, when foods are laid with sugar and salt, mimic responses that are in addicts of alcohol, cigarettes, and drugs often trigger the primitive neurochemical reward centers in the brain. While you assess your food mindfully, pay attention to the possible difference between the signs that your body desires and food because of its taste or health. Also, identify signs that show that you have developed a biological craving for it. It is possible for you to have a desire for a particular food for two reasons: because your body desires the nutrients in it or because you have developed a craving for the food.

Take note that when you assess your food, attention is not to be placed on the investigation of the calories, carbohydrates, fats, and salts that are allowed daily. If you focus on these aspects of your food, you will in no time be distracted from learning about the food accurately through direct experience. You should avoid choosing your food by the numbers. Choosing your food by the numbers involve you selecting what to eat by relying heavily on what you have read, and your computational skill rather than your senses. When a person eats by numbers, he or she will be concerned with the products he or she eats, and gets guidance from the diet claim, lasts fad, and from a medical expert. Well, it is quite great to follow the works of science and its recommendations; however, we should not rely solely on their information that we will let go or ignore our inner well of wisdom, which many people are presently guilty of. When you access the food that you want to eat mindfully, you would be in touch directly with the experience of the food itself and not on scientific calculations.

I remember my encounter with Regal. She explained that while she kept working on learning to assess her food, she discovered she began getting attracted to healthier and more natural foods. They became appealing to her senses more than the processed foods. When she stopped listening to her body mindfully, she discovered that her body did not respond well to nights of soda and pizza she had been used to. However, the nights she ate natural foods, such as broiled chicken and green beans with salad and watermelon, her body tended to respond differently. As she scanned through the plate of food, she discovered that all of her senses were engaged fully. She saw the colorfulness of the meal and the delicious smell of the watermelon. For her, the chicken filled her stomach with warmth and sustenance, while the taste of the green beans reminded her of the taste of the home-cooked meals of her childhood. When you give yourself to food assessment, you will become more sensitive to your body's desire to reject food before you eat it. After assessing your food by seeing and smelling it, you will create mindful attention to the taste of the food and its effect on your body. All of this will direct you on whether to keep eating or not. In the process of assessing your food, you may end up finding yourself making different food choices than you had ever made in the past.

CHAPTER EIGHT
SLOW DOWN THE PACE

The art of mindful eating requires taking each bite gradually without haste. When you slow down as you eat, your awareness of the moment when you are filled and able to satisfy your physical hunger's need will be activated. One way to enjoy your meal perfectly is to slow down. As I have mentioned earlier, you need to learn the art of mindful eating. Learning this art requires quite some conscious efforts from you as an individual. To achieve the best way of slowing down the pace as you eat, you should do the following:

- Pay attention to putting down your spoon (or fork) in between bites;

- Take a pause and a breath between bites;

- Chew your food thoroughly as you bite;

- When you try to talk and listen to others while

you drop your eating utensils constantly, pay attention to how the pace of your eating changes.

The importance of taking the aforementioned steps is for you to mindfully take in your food so as to be in charge of the food. When you observe your eating pace as you eat and pay attention to the food you are eating, you will get the best experience you want as you practice mindful eating.

WHY YOU NEED TO SLOW DOWN

You may be wondering if slowing down your eating pace has any significant effect on your eating. Well, the truth is, there are a lot of benefits to it. As much as it would help you achieve mindful eating, that alone is enough to explain to you the benefits you stand to gain by eating slowly. A study has revealed that when a person eats slowly, they tend to eat fewer calories and drink more water than they would have when they eat faster. Also, a person will likely feel less satisfied. More than the above, there are other benefits of slowing down the pace of your eating. One such is that it aids your ability to taste and savor your food. It may be difficult for most people to learn the process of slowing down as they eat. Remember, I mentioned earlier that it requires a conscious effort. You can ask yourself about the last time you ate your food, and you didn't even notice what you have eaten or how the food tasted. There are lots of reasons that can warrant the need to eat at such a speed that we will not even observe the taste of what we claimed to have eaten.

CHALLENGES TO SLOWING DOWN

There are certain circumstances that tend to make it a bit difficult and challenging to eat slowly. Such circumstances include being under time constraints when you share the table with other people and some environmental influences, such as loaded buffet tables. Also, if you are a nursing mother or someone who cares about the needs of children, you may find it difficult to have time for yourself to practice mindful eating or you may slow down the pace of your eating. You are likely to engage in eating often as you move from the kitchen to the table or within the compound. When you begin to pay attention to the rate at which you eat, you will begin to notice the rate at which the other people eat. It works as an eye-opener. Seeing people eating their food slowly will inspire you to stop eating fast.

Also, being accustomed to fast eating can be a hindrance. Some people are adept at doing whatever they need to get done as soon as possible. They usually do not want anything left for long, including eating. You would notice that such people move from one activity to another, from one task and meal to something else; as such, they are likely to want their plate empty and do something else. If you are guilty of this, you need to first pay attention to how you handle other activities and tasks given to you. Learn to slow down on other activities and don't take them in a swift manner. This step will help you learn how to slow down as you eat. The other activities include brushing your teeth, walking, driving, writing, or any other activities that you do daily. The more you slow down on other activities, the better it is for you to slow down as you eat mindfully.

HOW SLOW SHOULD YOU BE WHEN YOU EAT?

The possible question you may have is: how slow should you be as you eat? For every beginner, it is often said that the brain takes up to twenty minutes for it to register fully. Well, it is the truth, and it is quite bad for some of us who eat in less than twenty minutes and have even engaged in some other activities. Hence, if you are not carefully paying attention, you may end up filling yourself up as your brain catches up. When you slow down the pace, it will result in eating less, since the awareness of how filled you are will aid you to take a break. For every slow eater, you are already on the boulevard of mindful eating. The truth is, you already have this lesson under control. On the other hand, if you are a speed eater, you need to take the lesson seriously and check if you can slow down the pace at which you eat. I cannot say it will be easy to break the habit, but I know it is possible when you move in that direction.

CHAPTER NINE
INVESTIGATING YOUR HUNGER
AS YOU EAT

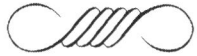

A nother lesson you need to learn in your journey of becoming a mindful eater is how to be aware of distractions and bring yourself back on track to tasting and assessing your hunger and level of satisfaction. You should investigate when you are halfway through with your eating. As you investigate, you will likely discover that you are no longer hungry, regardless of what you have left on your plate. As you eat, the investigation may reveal the answer the moment the food becomes less appealing. To effectively practice investigating your hunger as you eat, you need to stay away from unnecessary rules that expect you to finish your food. Instead, set up a choice in your mind to either stop or continue eating, depending on your hunger level. Having checked in with your hunger before you eat, you should further look into the level of your hunger as you keep eating to identify the best time for you to stop eating. As you eat, plan to stop halfway through the meal and observe your satisfaction level. Make the decision to stop eating once you are filled, no matter the taste of the food. While you investigate as you eat, you need to learn to do four things, which are:

- Learn to stop when you get halfway into your meal;

- Give yourself a deep breath;

- Look critically. Focus on the signs of satisfaction and taste of the food; and

- Keep eating the food if there is a need.

At the first move, you need to focus on your stomach in a mindful manner and identify your level using the hunger scale I identified above. Once you sense that you are satisfied, stop eating. However, if the hunger persists, you are permitted to keep eating. You should also try to ask yourself about the taste of the food. Look whether the food is worth your taste buds. Identify the motivating factor that is propelling you to keep eating. Are you eating because there is still food on your plate? The step you will take at the fourth stage will be determined by the information you get from your body and your taste buds. Investigating the hunger as you eat has proven to be effective for most people.

It is actually not easy to investigate your level of satisfaction and the taste of food. It is not as easy as it may look on paper. This is why you also need to be ready mentally and physically to make an effort. People tend to have two questions on the practice of investigating your hunger as you eat. The first is, how can a person know if he or she is satisfied?

The answer is that it is possible for a person to get filled up at the starting level. It is even possible for you to skip the satisfaction signals, and you end up becoming full. However, the truth you need to know is that there will always be a cue from your body that will convey to you the moment you need to stop eating. It is your duty to pay close attention. Listen closely and mindfully to the cues as you eat.

The second question is, why does a person keep eating even though he or she is satisfied?

Yes, it is possible for an individual to keep eating, even when he or she is filled. It is quite difficult for a person to stop eating in some situations. When a person eats after feeling satisfied, they are eating more than the hunger needs of their body. There are some reasons this happens to some people. Some of the reasons include:

1. **The Love for Food:** Some people love food as much as others love pets. When you love something, it is just expected of you to take your time with it. Similarly, people who like eating, especially when the food tastes so sweet, tend to overeat when they are filled. One thing you need to do in such a situation is to remember that you will always have access to more food in the future. There is an abundance of food for you. You can always get more to eat and fill your stomach some other time.

2. **The Fear of Hunger:** Many people are battling with the fear of the unknown. It often surprises me when someone says they are afraid of falling back to hunger again; hence, they will eat until fully satisfied. At times, people who were on a diet in the past often relapse into an obsession with food. The memory they keep with them about how they were restricted from taking certain food can lead them to seek all kinds of foods to devour. They often have the urge to want to eat so that they will not feel hungry. However, this affects mindful eating. One way to deal with the feeling from the past is to look into how you feel in the present. Attend to your thoughts and the effects of your past

conditioning mindfully and give yourself the assurance that there is food available for you anytime you need it. Also, it is possible for someone to pick up the attitude of fear of being hungry as a result of his or her childhood experience. Some people lived in a family where they were being fed at every point in time that they needed food, or even before they asked. Many mothers and grandmothers were so particular about feeding their children because they consider a child being full as the best way to be okay and safe. They perceive hunger as a source of discomfort and anxiety in certain situations. They had great intentions. However, their attitude built a dysfunctional method of experiencing hunger that affects a person's ability to practice mindful eating.

3. **Not Wanting to Waste the Food:** For some people, they are caught in the unempirical belief that they need to avoid wasting food, and as such, a person needs to clean their plate as they eat. People give excuses that it is wrong for you to waste your food. The money you are wasting, the number of people around you that are hungry, and many more. Often, this leads to a feeling of guilt in some people, and they find it

hard to throw food away. As a result, such people result in eating more than their capacities. This thought and the consequent result that it produces do not aid mindful eating practice.

Look inward and decide if how much you have eaten seems to be self-indulgent. It is often difficult to do. However, you need to understand that no matter how much you eat, you cannot solve the hunger problem in the world. Rather, you will end up doing yourself more evil than good. When a person eats too much, obesity will start stretching forth its hand of friendship, which you cannot easily reject. Regardless of the reason, you have to clean your plate; you need to find another means if truly you want to practice mindful eating. There are other means, such as serving yourself less or saving food for later. It might not have crossed your mind to take any step like this. However, it is part of the efforts you need to make if you want to achieve mindful eating. You can throw the food away; your stomach is not the wastebasket where you dump the food that you cannot eat. I tell you, there is no difference in putting unneeded food in your stomach or throwing it into the wastebasket. This requires you to pull down the stronghold of culture and beliefs that may try to tie you down in the process of practicing mindful eating.

INVESTIGATING YOUR HUNGER EFFECTIVELY

Socialization goes hand in hand with eating. However, engaging others in conversation is a great hindrance to mindful checking of your stomach. Talking to other people creates distractions, and this affects the possibility of you practicing mindful eating. When you are distracted, it will become difficult to check-in at the halfway point to investigate your hunger and satisfaction levels. As you eat with others, you need to pay attention to what you eat and your belly, if you must investigate your hunger. Avoid getting so much into the discussion that you will end up losing track of your hunger and end up filling yourself above the gauge.

You also have to pay attention to yourself more whenever you eat out in a restaurant. The reality of the restaurant is that you have control over the meal you request. However, you do not have the power over what the attendant serves you in terms of its quantity. The truth you need to understand is that they cook in the restaurant and do not have access to your hunger level while he or she serves you. Also, over the years, there has been an increase in the sizes of portions served by many cooks in restaurants. Therefore, you need to place your orders at the restaurants strategically. Make sure the quantity of the food is what you can finish alone. If that is not the case, then you need to get someone along who can share the food with you. You may take the remnant home if you are alone for you to eat later or probably throw it away. The most important thing is that you need to avoid overfeeding yourself. Investigating your hunger will be of help to you to understand how much food you need to place on your plate if you want to eat.

I remember someone asking me if it is okay to eat above the point of satisfaction. At times, it is possible to eat more than your biological hunger needs. You can take, for instance, you coming across new food that you have never eaten before. You can get the food and eat it despite the fact that you are already filled with your normal meal. And you will not get overfilled with eating the new food. Some situations, events, or circumstances may warrant you to take a quantity of food than you can actually take on a norm. In such instances, you will not regret your actions and not feel guilty.

The decision to stop eating often comes with a particular meal in question and the circumstances that surround the food. Advisably, you need to stop eating following the need of your hunger. The quantity of the food on your plate or the set down regulations in your culture, and any other beliefs, should not be the basis of your eating. Whenever you are eating feel that you are satisfied, you should stop. Train yourself consciously to know the right time to say yes and no. Mindfulness is meant to train you to have a say over your eating practice, and not to be controlled by any external factor.

CHAPTER TEN
CHEW THE FOOD THOROUGHLY

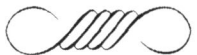

L
earning the art of mindful eating requires you to pay attention to how you chew your food. When you are focused on chewing, you will be paying attention to the varying sensations that are available to you. Also, you need to notice what happens to the food in your mouth as you keep on chewing. There is a different taste registered in your mouth. You also need to identify them, and as you identify, check if you enjoy the food or not. You should pay attention to the length of time it takes you to chew the food; that is one of the cores of mindful eating. While you are chewing your food, do you notice digestion happening immediately? And does your hunger keep fading away?

CHEWING EFFECTIVELY FOR MINDFUL EATING

For you to claim that you are practicing mindful

eating, you need to pay attention to your process of chewing the food in your mouth. Effective mindful eating is one that inculcates all the BASICS of mindful eating art. You have to be systematical with your food as you eat and pay close attention. By now, you are obviously aware that most lessons you need to learn for mindful eating require your attention; hence, you should not have challenges understanding the process of chewing your food as well. Chewing your food should be one bite by bite. You need to make sure that you bite your food thoroughly and move to the next bite as well. In the process of eating mindfully, your attention needs to be drawn toward the taste, sight, and smell of the food. You also need to give your time as you savor the food.

However, quite a large number of people have challenges slowing down on their food to appreciate all the things listed. The process of slowing down sometimes acts as an obstacle to learning mindful eating. Hence, you need to focus on the method that will empower you to infuse slowing down into your process of eating. By paying attention to how you chew the food, you are learning the art of slow and mindful eating. The secret of paying attention as you eat is that whatever we pay attention to often becomes meditation; hence, when you have a meditative experience as you chew your food, you tend to have a more extraordinary experience.

Lino Stanchich (1989) did a great deal of work on chewing by relating his father's story. His father was detained during the Second World War but survived the starvation diet that was served to him by thoroughly managing his process of chewing. Lino, himself ended up using the technique of chewing that his father taught him to survive during his detention in Yugoslavia. When a person chews gradually and thoroughly, there will likely be a reduction in the amount of food consumed by such a person. This is not far-fetched; as you chew gradually, you are mindfully savoring the food, and it will be quite easier for you to identify the level of your satisfaction as you eat. The thing is, you are not placed in the darkness and you will enjoy your meal as much as possible.

There have been others who offered explanations on mindful chewing like Lino. Horace Fletcher, also called *The Great Masticator* who was a great food enthusiast in the Victorian era, lived his life consistently that he gave certain tenets of eating to us before leaving. As recorded in Meriam Webster, his idea on mindful eating as recorded in Meriam Webster20110 bordered around, "eating when you are genuinely hungry, and not at the point of your anxiety, depression or when you are occupied; you can eat any food that appeals to your appetite, you should chew each bite of your food for up to thirty-two times or until the food gets dissolved; and you need to enjoy your food as you eat". In order to prove Fletcher's advice, some researchers took steps to test his doctrine on mindful chewing. Having compared the difference in the impacts of chewing the food for thirty-five times and ten times by a person, they discovered that by chewing the food longer, there is a reduction in the food intake level, regardless of the increase in the speed of chewing. Also, they discovered that when people eat faster, they eat lesser calories and have lower levels of the hormone ghrelin. The hormone ghrelin stimulates a person's appetite.

IMPORTANCE OF CHEWING THOROUGHLY

Chewing has a strong influence and power over you as you practice mindful eating. It may sound awkward or needless talking about paying attention to your process of food chewing. Nonetheless, the usefulness of chewing goes deep into your biological composition. Biologically, many processes are activated when you chew your food. Through the process of chewing, food particles are broken down into smaller pieces that the digestive enzymes can easily act on, lubricate, and make soft for it to become easily absorbable in your stomach for digestion. Chewing helps to reduce the challenge of constipation and acid reflux among many others. As you chew your food, your sense of taste will be activated. The activation of the sense of taste is what helps a person to decipher the nutrients and the potentially harmful toxic compounds in the food. As you chew your food, your mouth will take on the duty of a food processor. It enables you to gain more nutritional value and more energy from your food. By chewing your food mindfully, you will send signals to your brain, and that signal is what will register satisfaction in your brain. Also, the saliva that you produce as you eat will help to promote the health of your teeth. More to the importance of chewing thoroughly and mindfully is that it will help you to slow down; savor the taste of the meal, which is an important activity in the art of mindful eating.

CHAPTER ELEVEN
SAVORING THE FOOD WITH KNOWLEDGE

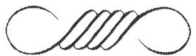

This is the last lap in the BASICS that you need to understand and follow to have complete knowledge of what it means for you to practice full mindful eating. To savor your food refers to carefully taking your time to select the food that you really like. At the same time, above your fondness of the food, you need to make your selection based on your satisfaction need at a point in time. The food you are choosing needs to honor your body and taste buds. To have a good experience of savoring your food, you need to be fully present for the mindful experience of eating, and you understand the pleasure you can get from it. Your attention needs to be on the sensations that you get from each bite that you take. Once you like it, you would experience the joy of savoring.

LEARNING TO SAVOR YOUR FOOD

MINDFULLY

To savor your food, you need first to choose the food that you like and will satisfy your taste and hunger need. You need to consider how you choose the food you want to eat. Are you taking a pause to have a reflection on the type of food or flavor that you think would satisfy your taste? Check if you are not eating what you see. Also, ascertain whether you are not eating out of habit or when you are distracted. Your selection of food should help you feel more satisfied when you are full. For some people, if they desire chocolate, they give in to it and eat it mindfully. However, some people tend to gaze at the chocolate and eat every other kind of food until they finally go back to the chocolate that triggered the hunger in the first place. The essence of your learning to savor is to identify what you eat for your taste and eat it mindfully. No amount of other meals can satiate your need for a specific food. If your taste and hunger seek a specific food, just go for it.

You can acquire the taste. When you give yourself to the eating of specific food over time, you will start developing a soft spot for such food and prefer the food's taste. So much so that you get used to eating all forms of sugary foods, fats, and processed foods. At a point in time, your taste will be dampened, and you would become used to the taste. The result is that you would prefer this form of eating than any other form. However, regardless of the taste you have right now, if you want to switch to another taste, you can always do that. Since you acquired the taste, you only need to let it go by unearning it through giving yourself to mindful eating with other great tastes. One thing about taking the step to change your taste for a specific kind of food is that you do not need to force the process of change. Whatever food it is that you can eat and savor mindfully, you can go for it. You do not need anyone to tell you to leave fast food behind. As you choose your food carefully, if you are tilted toward fast foods, you are free to go ahead and select them.

However, there is a way your taste senses can help you discover the need to go for more whole foods. Mindfully eating through savoring your food will show you the deficiencies in the processed foods you eat. Mindfulness helps to identify every artificial food and factors that affect the healthiness of the food that we eat. The process of savoring your meal will give you a whole body experience, which presents mindful eating as a holistic endeavor.

The reality is what I always love to live by. When you take too much fat, you will make your stomach feel queasy. Foods that are highly processed do not give you the satisfaction you need for long, and you cannot get the full energy you need to function throughout the whole day from it. Sugar has the propensity to make you get hungry and tired, and each time you eat foods filled with sugar, your brain will start experiencing difficulty to identify when you are full. When you eat whole foods, including vegetables, fruits, etc., your body will receive vitality and energy. Whole foods undergo a gradual process in the body and help to sustain you through the demands of the day. Pay attention to savoring your food mindfully, and you will notice how your food feels.

BE PRESENT WITH YOUR FOOD

The other step to take as you savor your food is to practice being present with your food and the pleasure that it has to offer you. Reversing every unconscious approach that you may have to food is possible. You only need to make yourself present as you savor the food. The taste of what you eat should be what will bring you back to the present. Being present refers to you being fully aware of the taste of the food you have before you. When your mind tries to wander off, call it back. As you taste the food, consider it an approach to reigning yourself in to be ever-present. You can always go back to the direct experience you get from taste repeatedly. When we rush to eat food, there is a high tendency that the taste will be lost, while a mindful process of savoring the same food will always prove to be the best way to enjoy its taste. We mostly have one thing or the other that demands our attention. However, as I have mentioned in the previous section on 'slow down the pace', you need to consciously learn to do things at a slower pace without rushing as it will help you achieve the perfect savoring you want to get at every point in time. The act of slowly savoring your food mindfully will make your experience being present with your food.

Distractions are powerful enough to block your sensitivity to the taste of the food that you have before you. However, each time you give yourself to mindful eating, you would end up discovering new information about your taste preferences be able to identify whether your body requires food or not. Always prepare your mind for whatever result you get after you have achieved being fully present with your food. There are three times for you in a day to experience a pleasant and mindful experience with the food that you take in. Learn to savor your food consistently, enjoy the sensation it gives, and the way it feels both in your mouth and body. When you learn to practice all the lessons in the BASICS acronym, you will experience an increase and improvement in the relationship that exists between you and the food you eat. At the same time, you would have an increase in your trust for your inner wisdom.

PART THREE

LIVING A MINDFUL EATING LIFESTYLE

CHAPTER TWELVE
FOLLOWING A FOUR-WEEK PLAN

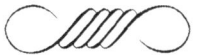

The practice of mindful eating requires time. It is a gradual process. If you have been an unconscious eater for over two, three, or more decades, teaching you a new approach to your habitual method of eating can be quite demanding and may seem difficult. However, taking conscious effort will help you achieve as much as you want to in the practice of mindful eating. To practice mindful eating, the lessons listed in the previous part of this book will be of help greatly. Below is a table that illustrates what you are expected to do in the four weeks of your engagement in learning to be adept at mindful eating. After the table, I have a broader explanation of what I have in the action that you need to take.

WEEKS	ACTION
One	Create awareness about mindful eating

Two	Build a habit around it
Three	Deal with external and inner factors that hinder mindful eating
Four	Start achieving your goal

- **Week One – Create an Awareness About Mindful Eating**

Living a life of mindful eating is not possible for a person that is not knowledgeable about it. The first step you need to take is to have a deep understanding of what mindful eating is all about. In the process, you are making yourself become aware of it and its importance. Understanding the importance and how you are expected to go about it is the awareness you need to create for you to start practicing mindful eating. More than that, you also need to identify your emotions. Before you start eating, identify your emotions and check if you are tense, depressed, tired, or anxious. Remember, you are not to eat because of any of these. When you eat as a result of anxiety, nervousness, stress, or fatigue, you are likely to overeat and fail at the first test of mindful eating.

Identifying the emotions that are dominant as you are about to eat will help you to avoid the possibility of you throwing yourself on your food without knowing. More so, creating awareness includes you having a deep knowledge around what you do at the table – being present as you eat. As you sit to wash your hands, you need to be aware of it. Also, part of you creating awareness includes you checking your breathing level. If it is shallow, you need to do away with it and start a mindful breathing technique, which is to be deep breathing. Your awareness of your breathing on the table in the first week will prevent you from being dominated at the table. The deep breathing practice should be done by swelling your abdomen. You also create awareness by activating your five senses in order to have a whole appreciation of all that you eat at every point in time. The color, the smell, shapes, textures, and even the shades of the taste need to be appreciated. Become aware of what your distractions are. Some elements work in such a way that they affect a person's approach to mindful eating. You need to identify those that are specifically working against you and deal with them rightly. The possible elements of distractions include radio, television, computer, your Smartphone, etc. The purpose of mindful eating is to make you enjoy every single bite of your meal and to give you a certain level of influence over your food. To achieve all these, you need to be aware of all these.

- **Week Two – Build a Habit Around It**

You need to dedicate the second week to creating a new habit of mindful eating. If you have been eating mindlessly, it is a habit that has been registered in you. To start eating mindfully, you need to make it a new habit by doing away with the old form that you are used to. As you create awareness around your table, start identifying the elements that can distract you and deal with them while you create a habit around it at the same time. The habit you need to create must make you become more aware of the table. You can start by slowing down with the process of brushing your teeth. That way, you would have curbed a wrong pattern of eating, like speed eating, and formed a new habit of slowly eating your food. Taking a slow shower or walking slow around the neighborhood are also ways to build a good habit of eating mindfully.

The purpose of forming a habit around mindful eating is to make you live in the moment as you eat without being carried away. You can adopt a little trick to making a habit out of mindful eating. A bracelet that tingles can be tied to your hand. Its sound is to call your attention back when you seem to wander away into negative thoughts. You may also breathe deeply between 2 and 3 times before you pick up a call. New habits are formed consistently. Achieving mindful eating involves you breathing deeply, assessing the food, slowing down the pace of your eating, investigating your hunger, chewing thoroughly, and savoring your meal. Give yourself to all of these. As you are presented with the next meal, you should give yourself to breathing rightly. You do not have to wait until you get to the table before you start observing your breathing. You may create time for yourself to observe and practice it; that way, it would become easier for you to practice it when it is time for you to eat.

Giving an assessment of the food can also be made a habit by consistently paying attention to other things around you. Do not pass by anything without carefully looking at its color, smell (if it has any), shapes, etc. This will create consciousness in you as you look into your food and hunger to assess it. The same rule goes for other lessons you learned in the BASICS of mindful eating. Do not wait until you start eating mindfully before you start practicing the act of investigation. You can investigate things around you to understand their status and how they are. This way, you would have become conversant with the act of investigation that it would become easier for you to exercise it as you eat. The second week is a week for you to make the lessons you have learned to become a part of you. Take note that you cannot make a habit in a week. The second week is starting the process. However, it continues until it becomes part of you.

- **Week Three – Deal with External and Inner Factors that Hinder Mindful Eating**

As you create awareness and build a habit around your purpose of practicing mindful eating, always remember that there are usually situations that are beyond the capacity that may have an effect on you. Some of the factors include stress from work or cravings for too many sweets or fats. There are lots of factors that hinder your possibility of achieving mindful eating. The best method you can utilize to combat the factors is meditation. Meditating for a few days will help you deal with every hindrance that may stop you from experiencing a complete mindful eating experience. You may schedule the meditation to occur at the same time of the day. It may be in the morning or in the evening, like after the day's work before going to bed. There are different guided meditations available on the internet; you may go for one to help you practice. Meditation will position you rightly by making you bring all your thoughts to a standpoint and clearing your mind of unwanted thoughts that may hinder you. During the meditation, you may sit on a chair and listen to what goes on inside you (you are simply checking for your emotions, thoughts, and possible tensions). You will also look at the outside factors, which are external, such as noise, smell, sounds, and so more. Remember, I mentioned earlier how taste could create a fondness in you for a specific food. You need to identify all that will stop you from practicing mindful eating fully and deal with it in a blow.

You may subscribe for more activities aside meditation to take care of your distractions. All you need to do is to be concentrated on your food as you eat. Hence, any activity that will give you concentration and make you learn the art of focusing will also suffice aside meditation. You may engage in gardening, walking, and some exercises, including deep breathing. You may also learn to eat by using your non-dominant hand. If you are used to your right hand, your left hand would be your non-dominant hand, and if you are used to your left hand, your right hand would be your non-dominant hand. Remember, you are changing your habit from being a mindless eater to being a mindful eater. The process requires you to change the direction of your brain to work in tandem; hence, changing your dominant hand at the table will help with this. The use of our hands is connected to the brain, and when we change it, the brain will sense it and conform.

- ## **Week Four – Start Achieving Your Goal**

You are welcome to the fourth week. At this time, if you have been following the steps in the previous three months, you need to take the advantages to embed in them and utilize the advantages to yourself. Achieving your goal involves you making the decision that you are ready for mindful eating. You do not have to wait until eternity before you start practicing it. Give yourself to eating mindfully by sitting at the table with the knowledge of the BASICS on your mind. Consciously breath at the table, assess the food, slow down intentionally, investigate your level of hunger and satisfaction, chew every bite carefully and thoroughly, and finally, savor every bite and enjoy every taste of the food. While you are at the table, you must be focused and pay attention as you eat. At least the first three mouthful bites you have should be taken consciously. When you are full, do not force it; but make an end and stop at the point. The goal is to eat mindfully, nothing more, nothing less; hence, consciously live out all the lessons you have learned from the last three weeks. Let your newly formed habit manifest as you eat, and you are on the boulevard of becoming an expert at mindful eating.

CHAPTER THIRTEEN
TRAINING YOUR CHILD TO
MINDFUL EATING

The reason most people eat mindlessly is not far-fetched. They have probably been indoctrinated into the act from childhood. We have many grown-up adults who eat the way they eat today as a result of how they were groomed to eat. Eating mindfully is best learned in childhood. At a tender age, every child has the propensity to learn faster and grasp whatever habit we need to make them have. It is often better for a person to grow with it because, as such, mindful eating would have become a crucial part of such a person. The tenets of mindfulness are a must-teach habit for every child to make them useful for himself or herself, and the family at large.

Mindfulness, also referred to as awareness, involves a person noticing his or her thoughts, feelings, bodily sensations, and the immediate environment without engaging in any form of judgment. When a child learns mindfulness, he or she would have been made to understand the importance of the present rather than going back to the past. You will not even look and be discouraged about the future that you are yet to see; rather, you would look at the thing in the NOW and make decisions based on what they portray. Mindfulness covers different aspects of a person's life. Your thinking, relationships, and eating are some of the instances of things you must pay attention to mindfully. The important element of mindfulness is that it is learned. As a parent that has built your mindfulness skills, it will be easier for you to teach your kids. And most importantly, it is often better to teach them as they grow so that your children will not have to experience a later knowledge of the importance of being mindful of what they eat and do.

WHY TEACH YOUR CHILD MINDFULNESS?

For whatever I want to do, I'm always asking myself the question, "Why?" I believe there needs to be a reason to delve into a particular activity or to learn a new thing. Whatever demands my time and efforts must be ready to give me the reason to engage in it. Training your children to practice mindfulness will have an effect on their ability to focus, especially in school. They will learn control over themselves and know how to calm down when they are upset. They will also learn to make decisions for themselves regardless of the situation. By teaching your child mindfulness, it will also apply to how he or she eats and improve the child's relationship with food. Just imagine how great it would be for a child to have a good relationship with food from childhood. Such a child would live above certain health conditions, such as obesity. There are three reasons people get to eat. These include physical hunger, emotional hunger, and the environment. The common type for most adults is emotional hunger. When you teach your child the intricacies of mindful eating, such a child would understand the difference that exists between the three types of hunger. The child will understand the effects of a certain level of food on themselves.

We eat to get energized and not be sick. However, many people eat to the extent that they feel sick and regret ever eating in the first place. This is the result of mindless eating. Mindful eating has a purpose that can be said in an expression: "That at the end of the meal, the person should feel physically better than he or she was before eating". Training your child the act of mindfulness in eating will help the child to recognize the specific feelings that are attached to their food and is sensation as they eat. They will have a full understanding of when stress, anxiety, depression, or any other external factors are requesting them to fill their stomachs with their biological hunger doing nothing about it. As a parent, you can easily reduce your stress daily by avoiding certain unpleasant health issues that may accompany eating mindlessly. I have seven steps you can take to train your child how to eat mindfully. They are as follows:

1. Utilize the Dr. Albers' Triple "S" model

The triple "S" model refers to Sit, Slow, and Savor. Just as every adult needs to observe this as they eat mindfully, you need to be conscious of your children as they eat. You would make sure that every moment at the table is geared toward making them better at eating by encouraging them to SIT while they are about to eat. Make sure he or she is not fast by making the child SLOW down the pace of his or her eating. The food needs to be savored to have a very detailed mindful experience; hence, make sure you SAVOR the food as well. It is common for kids to run around in the house while eating. This model is the best way to make them pay attention to what they eat and concentrate.

2. Create a Viable and Visible Location

Especially when it involves eating snacks, the location of the food matters a lot. Usually, we all want to eat fast foods. In this sense, anything that would not take much effort and time to prepare. Hence, if you want your child to have a mindful eating experience, it is best that you place every healthy and whole food in strategic locations where the child can easily locate it and take it to eat. Using a shelf or counter that a kid can reach would be helpful to achieve this. Make sure any food that would affect their process of practicing mindful eating is taken out of sight and promote the culture of mindful eating in your child.

3. You Can Proportion their Snacks in Small Bags

You should be the one deciding the number of snacks your kids take. When they come home, you should have a meal prepped proportional distribution of their snacks in a small bag that would curb their overeating of the snacks.

4. Make Food Become Fun

Kids are known for their fun-filled lifestyle. You should try to make their food become fun by arranging it in an alluring box. You can use 'the bento box' that is popularly used by kids in Japan. The bento box makes it possible to arrange food in an artistic form that will make the food looks like bugs, animals, and faces. When food becomes fun for children, they would not want it to end. Hence, the tendency to slow down, which is one of the basic tenets of the art of mindful eating.

5. Involve them in the Planning of their Meal

You can also make them have their input in the process of planning for their lunch. Make them actively involved in the planning and reviewing process of what they will have for lunch in the coming weeks. When they have an issue with any of the food for lunch, you can consider a new lunch in place of that which they do not like.

6. Always Keep Them Hydrated

As much as dehydration affects the adults, it also affects children. Thirst makes it seem like we are hungry. Get your child a water bottle that he or she can take around with them. At the same time, make sure you select a fun bottle that will engage them. The bottle should be filled with water, so they would have something to drink to stay hydrated.

7. Create Table Rule

Rules are one of the best methods you can use to bring children to order. Make sure that for every form of eating that would occur, it occurs on the table, even snacks. Many children enjoy eating while watching television. This is a source of distraction that easily affects mindful eating. Deal with this by stopping him or her and setting food at the table.

CONCLUSION
STAY AWAY FROM
MISCONCEPTIONS

The practice of mindful eating is demanding, no doubt. It has a lot of benefits at the same time, and this is why it has gained wide acceptance among many people. You should not be surprised to go out there and see people practicing mindful eating in the wrong way. The purpose of eating mindfully is to make you provide for your hunger needs and never leave the table the same as when you got there. You should not be someone who leaves sick from eating, but someone who leaves energized and having carefully chewed, savored, and slowly enjoyed the taste of the food. I have gathered a certain number of misconceptions that people have concerning mindful eating, and I will be debunking these myths. They are myths because they are not true of mindful eating practices. You cannot afford to drop this book and still have questions bothering you. If at all, it should be one that will enlighten you more, not a claim that is based on groundless rumors.

• Myth 1 – The Fad Based Myth

One popular misconception is that mindful eating is a temporal phenomenon that only stays for a while. Some people came up with the idea that it is only meant to serve a short-term purpose, after which it is no longer useful. As a result of this misconception, a lot of people are misusing mindful eating. They see it as a way of restricting their food intake. The error in this claim is that mindful eating is not a form of dieting. But people with this claim have made it become a diet. Mindful eating has come to stay. It does not depend on time for its relevance. It is, at the same time, sustainable. It is not teaching anyone to be restricted from his or her food selection. It is all concerned with being present with the moment. You give honor to your body and listen to its needs with care and kindness.

• Myth 2 – Mindful Eating Equates Healthy Living

They claim that when a person eats mindfully, he or she being healthy is not totally true. The essence of mindful eating is not to deal with any diseases or illnesses. It is only to make you pay attention to your food intake and identify the errors in it. Mindful eating helps you understand what it is that is happening in your body as you feed yourself. However, it does not equate healthiness. It helps you to identify the moment when you are filled and prevents you from filling yourself with food turned junks, which may get you sick. Mindfully eating is not a Keto diet that helps to deal with weight loss or seizures. You only gain the confidence that you have accurate knowledge concerning how you are feeling having eaten.

• Myth 3 – The Time Myth

Some people have challenges practicing mindfulness eating because they feel it takes time to eat mindfully, especially those who work in corporate organizations. They do not want anything to add into their schedules. However, mindful eating does not require any extra time from you whatsoever. Giving yourself to mindful eating will help you save more time because you are mindful of what you eat, and you will end up not eating what will likely give you any problem and demand a lot of your time afterward.

• Myth 4 – The Socialization Myth

Another common misconception by people is that

mindful eating does not go hand in hand with socialization. People claim they find it easy to be mindfully eating when they are alone, but they have difficulty when they are with people. They will always refer to the need for attention on them, and that requires a person to leave behind the other people. When you follow the basic steps you would take in achieving the art of mindful eating, you will discover that you need to eat slowly, and to do that, you need to make a pause in between bites by dropping your utensil. The best time for you to learn slowing down your pace of eating is now. More so, the importance of mindful eating does not lie in paying attention to what you eat. Instead, it is in your understanding of how you feel as you eat, and identifying the point of your satisfaction and when exactly it is that you need to eat more.

- **Myth 5 – The Weight Loss Myth**

There is a general claim that mindful eating helps deal with weight loss. There are few studies that have proven this. Their interests span from the need to provide a lasting solution to obesity. They are in search of a sustainable solution. However, the purpose of mindful eating is not losing weight. It is to make you have a good relationship with food, which can result in loss of weight. In some cases, some people gain weight while on mindful eating, while some people do not experience any changes in their weight.

• Myth 6 – The Quantity Myth

I call this the quantity myth because it has to do with the quantity of the food involved. Many people claim that mindful eating is all about a lesser amount of food, and this has made many people stay away from it. The claim is backed by saying that when a person pays attention to the satisfaction signals, he or she will notice the signal earlier than it should be. However, this claim just depicts one tenet of mindful eating. Mindful eating is to make you become non-judgmental about how much food you have to eat daily. As long as eating the food takes before you serve the purpose of your hunger's need, you should end the eating. There are times obviously that a person tends to feel hungry more; in such instance, you need to feed your biological hunger mindfully. Mindful eating is not about eating a low quantity of food; rather, it is about feeding yourself to the full level that you need to reach while you are mindful about it.

My barriers

- Emotional eating
- Recognising when I'm full
- Fear/anxiety/shame/guilt surrounding food.
- Eating too quickly
- Not drinking enough water.

Trigger foods:

- Chocolate anything
- Crisps
- Chips
- Anything potato
- Cheese

Printed in Great Britain
by Amazon